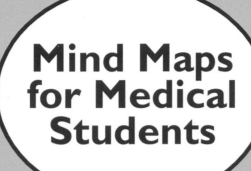

Mind Maps for Medical Students

T0132508

Mind Maps for Medical Students

SECOND EDITION

Olivia Smith

Core Surgical Trainee
Severn School of Surgery, UK

 CRC Press
Taylor & Francis Group
Boca Raton London New York

CRC Press is an imprint of the
Taylor & Francis Group, an **informa** business

Second edition published 2023
by CRC Press
6000 Broken Sound Parkway NW, Suite 300, Boca Raton, FL 33487-2742

and by CRC Press
4 Park Square, Milton Park, Abingdon, Oxon, OX14 4RN

CRC Press is an imprint of Taylor & Francis Group, LLC

ISBN: 9781032201146 (hbk)
ISBN: 9781032201122 (pbk)
ISBN: 9781003262275 (ebk)

DOI: 10.1201/9781003262275

Typeset in Linotype Frutiger LT Pro
by Evolution Design & Digital

In loving memory of my father D.J.W.Smith

Contents

How does one learn? This is the fundamental question for those who teach. To the student, however, 'How does one learn?' is the problem! This second edition of the successful *Mind Maps for Medical Students* is uniquely useful for both the teacher and student.

There seem to be a myriad of facts that fill the pages of textbooks – a myriad in each chapter! How does a student remember them, how does a student string them together to understand them and then finally recall them? In this era of booming knowledge and webs of digital connections, the volume of facts has become onerous.

In her time as an outstanding medical student at Hull York Medical School, Olivia used mind maps to create connections of knowledge and then taught this method to others. Her contributions led her to be runner up in 2016 for the 'Zeshan Qureshi Award for Outstanding Achievement in Medical Education'. Her books have been published in many languages internationally, including English, Chinese and Taiwanese. She has used this art in her research on quality of life in patients with complex abdominal wall hernias and complex abdominal wall reconstruction leading to an MD, as well as in revising and demonstrating surgical knowledge leading to successful completion of the MRCS examination.

Here, Olivia has gone back to the traditions of making the acquisition of facts simple, the connections organised and the recollection possible. Olivia's notes use mind maps – a powerful tool to aid understanding and recall while exploring myriad facts. These mind maps foster a skeleton upon which the reader can build a large body of knowledge.

I hope the readers of *Mind Maps for Medical Students* enjoy the layout and benefit from it. And that this book helps them explore the wonderful oceans of knowledge ahead. Happy surfing!

Chinta

Mr. Srinivas Chintapatla
Care Group Director – Cancer and Support Services
Consultant Surgeon (York Abdominal Wall Unit)
York Teaching Hospital NHS Foundation Trust

I am immensely grateful and humbled by the success of this book and the chance to provide a second edition. Acutely empathetic to the melancholies of medical training, it is my hope that this distillation of knowledge will help you in the intense preparation for your exams.

The book is an attempt to cover the main topics faced by medical students and presents these facts in a clear manner sufficient for final-year viva level. The work is not a substitute for larger, in-depth texts but it serves to complement them and act as an aide memoire to assist your understanding and revision.

It is not a definitive information source for students encountering a topic for the first time. However, it is a set of rapid revision notes covering a broad range of medical topics, ideally suited to students and early postgraduates revising for exams. This distillation of knowledge will save many hours of note-taking for other students. The format will appeal to those who construct their knowledge in logical sequences and the layout will allow the reader to add notes and annotations as information changes or to add a local context.

I hope that you enjoy this book and wish you all the very best of luck in your examinations and career.

Olivia Smith
MBBS(Hons), BSc(Hons), MSc(Dist), MD, PGcert, MRCS(Eng)
Core Surgical Trainee, Severn School of Surgery, UK

5-ASA	5-aminosalicylic acid
ABG	arterial blood gas
ACE	angiotensin converting enzyme
ACE-i	angiotensin converting enzyme inhibitor
ACE-III	Addenbrooke's Cognitive Examination
ACTH	adrenocorticotrophic hormone
ADH	antidiuretic hormone
ADL	activity of daily living
ADP	adenosine diphosphate
ADPKD	autosomal dominant polycystic kidney disease
AF	atrial fibrillation
Ag	antigen
AIDS	acquired immunodeficiency syndrome
AKI	acute kidney injury
ALL	acute lymphoblastic leukaemia
ALP	alkaline phosphatase
AML	acute myeloid leukaemia
ANA	antinuclear antibody
ANCA	antineutrophil cytoplasmic antibody
APLA	antiphospholipid antibody
APML	acute promyelocytic leukaemia
Apo	apolipoprotein
APP	amyloid precursor protein
APTT	activated partial thromboplastin time
ARB	angiotensin receptor blocker
ARDS	acute respiratory distress syndrome
ARPKD	autosomal recessive polycystic kidney disease
ARR	aldosterone:renin ratio
ART	antiretroviral therapy
ASD	atrial septal defect
ATP	adenosine triphosphate
ATRA	all-trans retinoic acid
AV	atrioventricular
BBB	blood–brain barrier
BMI	body mass index
BNP	brain natriuretic peptide
BP	blood pressure
BPH	benign prostatic hypertrophy
CABG	coronary artery bypass graft
CADASIL	cerebral autosomal dominant arteriopathy with subcortical infarcts and leukoencephalopathy
CAPS	catastrophic antiphospholipid syndrome
CCP	cyclic citrullinated peptide
CD	cluster of differentiation
CEA	carcinoembryonic antigen
CHF	congestive heart failure
CJD	Creutzfeldt–Jakob disease
CKI	chronic kidney injury
CLL	chronic lymphocytic leukaemia
CML	chronic myeloid leukaemia
CMV	cytomegalovirus
CNS	central nervous system
COPD	chronic obstructive pulmonary disease
COX	cyclooxygenase
CRC	colorectal cancer
CREST	Calcinosis, Raynaud's disease, oEsophageal dysmotility, Sclerodactyly and Telangiectasia
CRP	C-reactive protein
CSF	cerebrospinal fluid
CT	computed tomography
CTA	computed tomography angiogram

CTS	carpal tunnel syndrome	**ESKD**	end-stage kidney disease
CVS	chorionic villus sampling	**ESR**	erythrocyte sedimentation rate
CXR	chest X-ray		
DaTSCAN	ioflupane ^{123}I for injection	**ESWL**	extracorporeal shock wave lithotripsy
DCIS	ductal carcinoma in situ		
DEXA	dual-energy X-ray scan	**FAP**	familial adenomatous polyposis
DFA	direct fluorescent antibody test		
		FBC	full blood count
DHT	dihydrotestosterone	**FEV$_1$**	forced expiratory volume
DI	diabetes insipidus	**FFP**	fresh frozen plasma
DIC	disseminated intravascular coagulation	**FISH**	fluorescence in situ hybridisation
DIP	distal interphalangeal (joint)	**FNA**	fine needle aspiration
DLCO	diffusing capacity of the lung for carbon monoxide	**FRC**	functional residual capacity
		FSH	follicle-stimulating hormone
DM	diabetes mellitus	**FTA**	fluorescent treponemal antibody absorption
DMARD	disease modifying antirheumatic drug		
		FVC	forced vital capacity
DNA	deoxyribonucleic acid	**GABA**	gamma-aminobutyric acid
DPP	dipeptidyl peptidase	**GBM**	glomerular basement membrane
DVLA	Driver and Vehicle Licensing Agency		
		(c)GFR	(calculated) glomerular filtration rate
DVT	deep vein thrombosis		
DWI	diffusion-weighted MRI	**GH**	growth hormone
EBV	Epstein–Barr virus	**GHRH**	growth hormone-releasing hormone
ECG	electrocardiography		
ECHO	echocardiography	**GI**	gastrointestinal
EEG	electroencephalography	**GIT**	gastrointestinal tract
EIA	enzyme immunoassay	**GLP**	glucagon-like peptide
ELISA	enzyme linked immunosorbent assay	**GnRH**	gonadotrophin-releasing hormone
		GORD	gastro-oesophageal reflux disease
EMA	eosin-5'-maleimide		
EMB	eosin methylene blue	**Gp**	glycoprotein
EMG	electromyography	**G6PD**	glucose-6-phosphate dehydrogenase
ENA	extractable nuclear antigen		
EPEC	enteropathogenic *E. coli*	**GTN**	glyceryl trinitrate
EPO	erythropoietin	**HAV**	hepatitis A virus
ERCP	endoscopic retrograde cholangiopancreatography	**Hb**	haemoglobin
		HbA1c	glycated haemoglobin
ERV	expiratory reserve volume		

HBV	hepatitis B virus	LAMA	long-acting muscarinic antagonist
HCC	hepatocellular carcinoma	LBBB	left bundle branch block
Hct	haematocrit	LDH	lactate dehydrogenase
HCV	hepatitis C virus	LFTs	liver function tests
HDV	hepatitis D virus	LH	luteinising hormone
HELLP	Haemolysis, Elevated Liver enzymes and Low Platelets	LHRH	luteinising hormone-releasing hormone
HEV	hepatitis E virus	LMN	lower motor neuron
HGPRT	hypoxanthine–guanine phosphoribosyltransferase	LMWH	low molecular weight heparin
HHV	human herpes virus	LP	lumbar puncture
HIV	human immunodeficiency virus	LTRA	leukotriene receptor antagonists
HNPCC	hereditary nonpolyposis colorectal cancer	LVF	left ventricular failure
HPV	human papilloma virus	MALT	mucosa-associated lymphoid tissue (lymphoma)
HRT	hormone replacement therapy	MAO	monoamine oxidase
HS	hereditary spherocytosis	MCH	mean corpuscular haemoglobin
HTLV-1	human T-lymphotrophic virus-1	MCPJ	metacarpophalangeal joint
HUS	haemolytic–uraemic syndrome	MCV	mean corpuscular volume
IBD	inflammatory bowel disease	MDT	multidisciplinary team
IBS	irritable bowel syndrome	MDS	myelodysplastic syndromes
ICS	inhaled corticosteroid	MEN	multiple endocrine neoplasia (syndrome)
ICU	intensive care unit		
IFA	immunofluorescence assay	MI	myocardial infarction
IFN	interferon	MLCK	myosin light chain kinase
Ig	immunoglobulin	MMR	mumps, measles, rubella
IGF	insulin-like growth factor	MND	motor neuron disease
IL	interleukin	MRA	magnetic resonance angiogram
INR	international normalised ratio		
IPSS	International Prostate Symptom Score	MRCP	magnetic resonance cholangiopancreatography
IRV	inspiratory reserve volume	MRI	magnetic resonance imaging
IV	intravenous	MS	multiple sclerosis
IVU	intravenous urogram	MSK	musculoskeletal
JVP	jugular venous pressure	MTPJ	metatarsophalangeal joint
KUB	kidney, ureter, bladder	NAAT	nucleic acid amplification test
LABA	long-acting beta-agonist	NBM	nil by mouth

NICE	National Institute for Health and Care Excellence	**PT**	prothrombin time
NMDA	N-methyl-D-aspartate	**PTH**	parathyroid hormone
NPI	Nottingham Prognostic Index	**PTT**	partial thromboplastin time
NSAID	nonsteroidal anti-inflammatory drug	**RA**	rheumatoid arthritis
		RAAS	renin–angiotensin–aldosterone system
NSCC	non-small cell carcinoma	**RBC**	red blood cell
NSTEMI	non-ST elevation myocardial infarction	**RCC**	renal cell carcinoma
		RCS	Raynaud Condition Score
OA	osteoarthritis	**RDS**	respiratory distress syndrome
OCP	oral contraceptive pill	**RNA**	ribonucleic acid
OGD	oesophago-gastro-duodenoscopy	**RPR**	rapid plasma regain
		RV	residual volume
OPSI	overwhelming post-splenectomy infection	**RVF**	right ventricular failure
		SABA	short-acting beta-agonist
PaCO₂	arterial partial pressure of carbon dioxide	**SAMA**	short-acting muscarinic antagonist
PaO₂	arterial partial pressure of oxygen	**SCC**	small cell carcinoma
		SERM	selective oestrogen receptor modulator
PAH	phenylalanine hydroxylase		
PAS	periodic acid stain	**SIADH**	syndrome of inappropriate antidiuretic hormone secretion
PCI	percutaneous coronary intervention		
PCNL	percutaneous nephrolithotomy	**SLE**	systemic lupus erythematosus
		SPECT	single photon emission computed tomography
PCR	polymerase chain reaction		
PE	pulmonary embolus	**SSRI**	selective serotonin reuptake inhibitor
PEP	post-exposure prophylaxis		
PET	positron emission tomography	**STEMI**	ST elevation myocardial infarction
PG	prostaglandin		
PI	protease inhibitor	**STI**	sexually transmitted infection
PIP	proximal interphalangeal	**SUDEP**	sudden unexplained death in epilepsy
PL	phospholipid		
PMR	polymyalgia rheumatica	**SWL**	shockwave lithotripsy
PPAR	peroxisome proliferator-activated receptor	**T₃**	triiodothyronine
		T₄	thyroxine
PPI	proton pump inhibitor	**TB**	tuberculosis
PR	per rectum	**TdT**	terminal deoxynucleotidyltransferase
PSA	prostate specific antigen		

TCC	transitional cell carcinoma	**U&Es**	urine and electrolytes
TFTs	thyroid function tests	**UMN**	upper motor neuron
TIA	transient ischaemic attack	**UPEC**	uropathogenic *E. coli*
TIBC	total iron binding capacity	**USS**	(abdominal) ultrasound scan
TLC	total lung capacity	**URS**	ureteroscopy
TNF	tumour necrosis factor	**UTI**	urinary tract infection
ToF	tetralogy of Fallot	**VC**	vital capacity
TPHA	*Treponema pallidum* haemagglutination test	**VEP**	visual evoked potential
TPPA	*Treponema pallidum* particle agglutination test	**VDRL**	Venereal Disease Research Laboratory
TSH	thyroid-stimulating hormone	**V/Q**	ventilation/perfusion
TURP	transurethral resection of the prostate	**VSD**	ventricular septal defect
		VWF	von Willebrand factor
TV	tidal volume	**VZV**	varicella-zoster virus
		WCC	white cell count

Map 1.1 Heart Failure

Classification

Framingham Criteria for Congestive Heart Failure: 2 major criteria *or* 1 major criteria and 2 minor criteria:

- Major criteria: **PAINS**
  ○ **P**aroxysmal nocturnal dyspnoea.
  ○ **A**cute pulmonary oedema.
  ○ **I**ncreased heart size, Increased central venous pressure.
  ○ **N**eck vein dilation.
  ○ **S**3 gallop.
- Minor criteria: **PAIN**
  ○ **P**leural effusion.
  ○ **A**nkle oedema (bilateral).
  ○ **I**ncreased heart rate >120 beats/min.
  ○ **N**octurnal cough.

New York Heart Association Classification for Heart Failure

I: No limitation of physical activity.
II: Slight limitation of physical activity.
III: Marked limitation of physical activity.
IV: Inability to carry out physical activity.

Causes

Anything that causes myocardial damage may lead to heart failure.
Examples include:

- Coronary artery disease.
- Hypertension.
- Atrial fibrillation.
- Valve disease.
- Cardiomyopathies.
- Infective endocarditis.
- Anaemia.
- Endocrine disorders.
- Cor pulmonale: this is right ventricular failure secondary to pulmonary disease.

What is heart failure?

This may be defined as the inability of cardiac output to meet the physiological demands of the body. It can be classified in several ways:

- Left ventricular failure (LVF): symptoms of LVF: paroxysmal nocturnal dyspnoea, wheeze, nocturnal cough with pink sputum caused by pulmonary oedema.
- Right ventricular failure (RVF): symptoms of RVF, which is usually caused by LVF or lung disease, peripheral oedema and ascites.
- Low output and high output heart failure. This is due to excessive afterload, excessive preload or pump failure.

Pathophysiology

See page 4.

MAP 1.1 Heart Failure

Treatment

- Conservative: smoking cessation advice, weight loss, promotion of healthy diet and exercise.
- Medical: ACE-i (can be offered first line) at low dose and titrate upwards as tolerated. Do not give to those who have valvular disease until they have been assessed by a specialist. ARB is an alternative to ACE-i if ACE-i is not tolerated. Diuretics, e.g. furosemide/spironolactone, may be given to provide relief from overload.
  - Consider prescribing an antiplatelet to people with atherosclerotic arterial disease (including coronary heart disease).
    - Consider statin therapy after CVD risk assessment.
    - Refer for supervised exercise-based group rehabilitation programme for people with heart failure.
    - Offer annual flu vaccine and once-only pneumococcal vaccine.
  - The following specialist treatments may be initiated after specialist assessment:
    - Combination of loop and thiazide diuretic.
    - Aldosterone antagonist (spironolactone or eplerenone).
    - Sacubitril valsartan.
    - Hydralazine in combination with a nitrate (especially if the person is of African–Caribbean origin).
    - Digoxin.
    - Ivabradine (slows the heart rate in sinus rhythm).
    - Anticoagulation may be indicated for people with heart failure who are in sinus rhythm and have a history of thromboembolism, left ventricular aneurysm or intracardiac thrombus.
    - Intravenous iron.
- Surgical intervention:
  - Cardiac resynchronisation therapy.
  - Insertion of an implantable cardioverter defibrillator (ICD).
  - Coronary revascularisation.
  - Cardiac transplantation.

Complications

- Arrhythmia.
- Valve dysfunction.
- Renal failure.
- Liver failure.
- Stroke.

Investigations

- Bloods:
  - FBC, U&Es, LFTs, TFTs, lipid profile.
  - BNP (brain natriuretic peptide). It suggests how much the myocytes are stretched. BNP is arguably cardioprotective as it causes Na^+ ion and H_2O excretion in addition to vasodilation. A concentration >400 pg/mL (>116 pmol/L) is suggestive of heart failure.
- CXR: **ABCDE**
  - **A**lveolar oedema.
  - Kerley **B** lines.
  - **C**ardiomegaly.
  - **D**ilated upper lobe vessels.
  - pleural **E**ffusion.
- ECHO: look for ejection fraction, valve disease and regional wall motion abnormalities.
- ECG.

Map 1.2 Pathophysiology of Congestive Heart Failure (CHF)

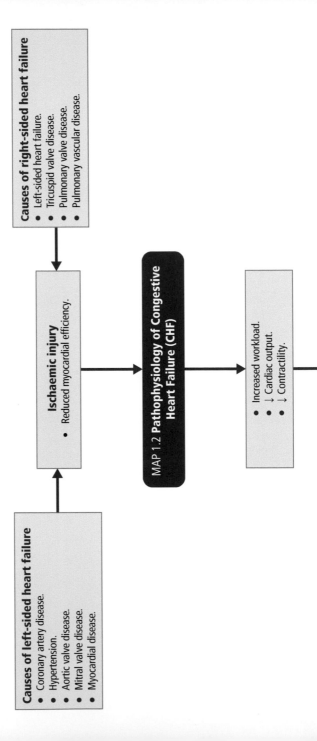

Causes of right-sided heart failure
- Left-sided heart failure.
- Tricuspid valve disease.
- Pulmonary valve disease.
- Pulmonary vascular disease.

Causes of left-sided heart failure
- Coronary artery disease.
- Hypertension.
- Aortic valve disease.
- Mitral valve disease.
- Myocardial disease.

Ischaemic injury
- Reduced myocardial efficiency.

MAP 1.2 **Pathophysiology of Congestive Heart Failure (CHF)**

- Increased workload.
- ↓ Cardiac output.
- ↓ Contractility.

Activates compensatory mechanisms

- Activation of the renin–angiotensin–aldosterone system (RAAS) causes Na^+ ion and H_2O retention, and peripheral vasoconstriction. This increases preload.
- Activation of the sympathetic nervous system increases heart rate and causes peripheral vasoconstriction. This increases afterload.
- ↑ Myocyte size.

Chronic activation of these compensatory mechanisms worsens heart failure and leads to increased cardiac damage.

Remember that:

- The cause of cardiac dilation is increased end-diastolic volume.
- The raised jugular venous pressure (JVP) is related to right-sided heart failure and fluid overload.
- Hepatomegaly is caused by congestion of the hepatic portal circulation.

Investigations

- ECG: this may show:
  - ST elevation, ST depression, inverted T waves.
  - New left bundle branch block (LBBB).
  - Pathological Q waves.
- CXR: this may show:
  - Cardiomegaly.
  - Pulmonary oedema.
  - Widening of the mediastinum.
- Bloods: look for cardiac biomarkers:
  - Troponin I.
  - Troponin T.
- Angiography with the view to performing percutaneous coronary intervention (PCI).

Pathophysiology

See page 9 for the pathophysiology of atherosclerosis.

Type of infarct

- Transmural:
  - Affects all of the myocardial wall.
  - ST elevation and Q waves.
- Subendocardial:
  - Necrosis of <50% of the myocardial wall.
  - ST depression.

**MAP 1.3
Myocardial Infarction (MI)**

What is MI?

Also known as a heart attack. It occurs when there is myocardial necrosis following atherosclerotic plaque rupture, which occludes one or more of the coronary arteries. MI is part of the acute coronary syndromes. The acute coronary syndromes comprise:

- ST elevation MI (STEMI).
- Non-ST elevation MI (NSTEMI).
- Unstable angina.

Causes

- Type 1 MI – a primary coronary arterial event due to atherosclerosis.
- Type 2 MI – secondary to an imbalance in myocardial oxygen supply and demand without atherothrombosis, e.g. severe anaemia, coronary artery spasm.

Symptoms

- Nausea, sweating, palpitations.
- Crushing chest pain for more than 20 minutes.
- Pain radiating down left arm or into the jaw.
- Epigastric pain that is severe and may be mistaken for reflux or another upper gastrointestinal problem.
- N.B. Can be silent in diabetics.

Signs

Remember these as **RIP**:

- **R**aised jugular venous pressure (JVP).
- **I**ncreased pulse, blood pressure changes.
- **P**allor, anxiety.

Treatment

- Conservative: lifestyle measures such as smoking cessation and increased exercise.
- Medical – **MONA B** for immediate management:
  - **M**orphine.
  - **O**xygen (if hypoxic).
  - **N**itrates (glyceryl trinitrate [GTN]).
  - **A**nticoagulants, e.g. aspirin and an antiemetic.
  - **B**eta-blockers if no contraindication.

On discharge all patients should be prescribed: aspirin, an angiotensin converting enzyme (ACE) inhibitor, a beta-blocker (if no contraindication; calcium channel blockers are good alternatives) and a statin.

- Surgical: reperfusion with PCI if STEMI. PCI may also be used in NSTEMI but if NSTEMI patients are not having immediate PCI, fondaparinux (a factor Xa inhibitor) or a low molecular weight heparin (LMWH) may be given subcutaneously.

Complications

- Cardiogenic shock, Cardiac arrhythmia.

N.B. Atrial fibrillation (AF) increases a patient's risk of stroke. AF presents with an irregularly irregular pulse and an ECG with absent P waves, irregular RR intervals, an undulating baseline and narrow QRS complexes. Consider starting anticoagulation therapy in line with local hospital guidelines and in context with tools such as the HAS-BLED score, which estimates risk of major bleeding for patients on anticoagulation to assess risk–benefit in atrial fibrillation care.

- Pericarditis.
- Emboli.
- Aneurysm formation.
- Rupture of ventricle.
- Dressler's syndrome: an autoimmune pericarditis that develops 2–10 weeks post MI. This is a triad of: 1) fever; 2) pleuritic pain; 3) pericardial effusion.
- Rupture of free wall.
- Papillary muscle rupture.
- Sudden death.
- Hypertension.
- Ventricular septal defect.
- Frozen shoulder and shoulder–hand syndrome.

Map 1.4 Angina Pectoris

What is angina pectoris?

Angina pectoris may be defined as substernal discomfort that is precipitated by exercise but relieved by rest or GTN spray.

Causes

- Atherosclerosis.
- Rarely anaemia and tachyarrhythmia.

Precipitants

- Exercise.
- Cold weather.
- Heavy meals.

Types of angina

- Stable angina: precipitated by exercise but relieved by rest.
  ST DEPRESSION
- Unstable angina: pain at rest, worsening symptoms.
  ST DEPRESSION
- Decubitus angina: triggered by lying flat.
  ST DEPRESSION
- Prinzmetal angina: due to coronary artery spasm.
  ST ELEVATION

Investigations: ECG

- ECG for signs of ST depression or ST elevation. Exercise ECG is no longer recommended by NICE guidelines.
- **C**T scan, **C**oronary **C**alcium Score (this is measured on CT) and Coronary angiography.
- **G**o for thallium scan.

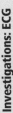

MAP 1.4 **Angina Pectoris**

Pathophysiology of atherosclerosis

Atherosclerosis is a slowly progressive disease and is the underlying cause of ischaemic heart disease when it occurs in the coronary arteries.

There are 3 stages of atheroma formation:

1 Fatty streak formation

Lipids are deposited in the intimal layer of the artery. This, coupled with vascular injury, causes inflammation, increased permeability and white blood cell recruitment. Macrophages phagocytose the lipid and become foam cells. These form the fatty streak.

2 Fibrolipid plaque formation

Lipid within the intimal layer stimulates the formation of fibrocollagenous tissue. This eventually causes thinning of the muscular media.

3 Complicated atheroma

This occurs when the plaque is extensive and prone to rupture. The plaque may be calcified due to lipid acquisition of calcium. Rupture activates clot formation and thrombosis. If the coronary artery is partially occluded the result is myocardial ischaemia and therefore angina. If the coronary artery is completely occluded then the result is myocardial necrosis and MI.

Complications

- MI.
- Stroke.

Treatment

- Conservative: modify risk factors, e.g. control cholesterol, control diabetes, smoking cessation advice, weight loss, increase exercise and control hypertension.
  Identification of patients who are at risk, e.g. using QRisk score.
- Medical:
  - Nitrates: glyceryl trinitrate (GTN) spray. Side effects include headache and hypotension.
  - **A** – Aspirin.
  - **B** – Beta-blockers but contraindicated in asthma and chronic obstructive pulmonary disease (COPD).
  - **C** – Ca²⁺ antagonists especially if beta-blockers are contraindicated.
  - K⁺ channel activator, e.g. nicorandil.
- Surgery: percutaneous transluminal coronary angioplasty or coronary artery bypass graft (CABG).

Map 1.5 Infective Endocarditis

Classification of infective endocarditis

Duke criteria: 2 major criteria *or* 1 major and 3 minor criteria *or* 5 minor criteria.

- Major criteria:
  - ○ 2 separate positive blood cultures.
  - ○ Endocardial involvement.
- Minor criteria: **FIVE**
  - ○ **F**ever >38°C.
  - ○ **I**V drug user or predisposing heart condition, and
  - ○ **I**mmunological phenomena, e.g. Osler's nodes or Roth's spots.
  - ○ **V**ascular phenomena, e.g. mycotic aneurysm or Janeway lesions.
  - ○ **E**chocardiograph findings.

Pathophysiology

Infective endocarditis is a rare infection that usually affects patients who already have a structural valve abnormality.

The reason why heart valves are targeted is because the valves of the heart have limited blood supply and consequently white blood cells cannot reach the valves through the blood. Circulating bacteria adhere to the valve causing vegetations.

What is infective endocarditis?

It is an infection of the endocardium usually involving the heart valves, with 'vegetation' of the infectious agent.

The mitral valve is more commonly affected but the tricuspid valve is implicated in IV drug users.

Risk factors

- IV drug abuse.
- Cardiac lesions.
- Rheumatic heart disease.
- Dental treatment: requires antibiotic prophylaxis.

Investigations

- Blood cultures: take 3 separate cultures from 3 peripheral sites.
- Bloods for anaemia.
- Urinalysis; microscopic haematuria.
- CXR.
- Transoesophageal/transthoracic ECHO for vegetations.

Causative agents

- *Streptococcus viridans*.
- *Staphylococcus aureus*.
- *Staphylococcus epidermidis*.
- Diphtheroids.
- Microaerophilic streptococci.
- HACEK group: *Haemophilus, Actinobacillus, Cardiobacterium, Eikenella* and *Kingella*.

MAP 1.5 Infective Endocarditis

Signs and symptoms

Remember this as **FROM JANE:**

- **F**ever.
- **R**oth's spots (seen on fundoscopy).
- **O**sler's nodes (painful nodules seen on the fingers and toes).
- new **M**urmur.

- **J**aneway lesions (painless papules seen on the palms and plantars).
- **A**naemia.
- **N**ails: splinter haemorrhages.
- **E**mboli.

FIGURE 1.1 Heart Valves

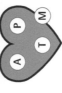

Remember the heart valves as:
All Prostitutes Take Money
(Aortic, Pulmonary, Tricuspid, Mitral).

Treatment

Depends on the causative agent. Check hospital antibiotic guidelines.

- Conservative: maintain good oral hygiene.
- Medical: follow local trust antibiotic prescribing policy but some examples of empirical therapy include **benzylpenicillin** and **gentamicin.**
  - Streptococci: **benzylpenicillin** and **amoxicillin.**
  - Staphylococci: **flucloxacillin** and **gentamicin.**
  - *Aspergillus*: **miconazole.**
- Surgical: valve repair or valve replacement.

Complications

- Heart failure.
- Arrhythmias.
- Abscess formation in the cardiac muscle.
- Emboli formation: may cause stroke, vision loss or spread the infection to other regions of the body.

Table 1.1 Aortic Valve Disease

TABLE 1.1 Aortic Valve Disease

Valve lesion	Causes	Symptoms	Signs	Murmur	Investigations	Treatment	Complications
Aortic stenosis	Atherosclerotic-like calcific degeneration Congenital bicuspid valve Rheumatic heart disease	Syncope Dyspnoea Angina	Narrow pulse pressure Slow rising pulse	Crescendo-decrescendo ejection systolic murmur, which radiates to the carotids	ECG: left ventricular hypertrophy; AV block CXR: poststenotic dilation of the ascending aorta; may see calcification of valve on lateral view ECHO: confirms diagnosis; allows severity and valve area to be assessed	Conservative: manage cardiovascular risk factors, e.g. smoking cessation Medical: manage cardiovascular risk factors, e.g. control blood pressure Surgical: valve replacement is the treatment of choice	Sudden death Arrhythmia Heart failure Infective endocarditis
Aortic regurgitation	**Acute** Cusp rupture Connective tissue disorders, e.g. Marfan's syndrome	Dyspnoea Angina Heart failure	Waterhammer pulse Wide pulse pressure	Decrescendo early diastolic murmur	ECG: left ventricular hypertrophy	Conservative: manage cardiovascular risk factors, e.g. smoking cessation	Heart failure Arrhythmia Infective endocarditis

Aortic dissection Perforation secondary to infection **Chronic** Rheumatoid arthritis Ankylosing spondylitis Syphilis	Traube's sign: a 'pistol shot' heard over the femoral artery De Musset's sign: head nodding in time with heart beat Quincke's sign: pulse felt in the nail Signs of systemic disease	CXR: may see cardiomegaly and pulmonary oedema if patient has heart failure ECHO: confirms diagnosis; allows severity and aortic root to be assessed	Medical: manage heart failure by following NICE guidelines Surgical: valve replacement is the treatment of choice

Table 1.1 Aortic Valve Disease

Table 1.2 Mitral Valve Disease

TABLE 1.2 **Mitral Valve Disease**

Valve lesion	Causes	Symptoms	Signs	Murmur	Investigations	Treatment	Complications
Mitral stenosis	Rheumatic heart disease Calcification of valve Rheumatoid arthritis Ankylosing spondylitis Systemic lupus erythematosus (SLE) Malignant carcinoid	Dyspnoea Palpitations if in atrial fibrillation (AF) Heart failure Haemoptysis	Malar flush Tapping apex beat Hoarse voice (Ortner's syndrome) Irregularly irregular pulse if in AF	Low pitch mid-diastolic murmur with opening snap	ECG: atrial fibrillation; bifid P waves CXR: pulmonary oedema and enlarged left atrium may be seen ECHO: confirms diagnosis; allows severity and valve area to be assessed	Conservative: manage cardiovascular risk factors, e.g. smoking cessation Medical: manage AF and heart failure by following NICE guidelines Surgical: valve replacement is the treatment of choice	AF Heart failure Infective endocarditis
Mitral regurgitation	Rheumatic heart disease Papillary muscle rupture Infective endocarditis Prolapse	Dyspnoea Palpitations if in AF Heart failure Symptoms of infective endocarditis	Irregularly irregular pulse if in AF Displaced apex beat	A harsh pansystolic murmur radiating to the axilla	ECG: atrial fibrillation; bifid P waves CXR: may see cardiomegaly and pulmonary oedema if patient has heart failure	Conservative: manage cardiovascular risk factors, e.g. smoking cessation	AF Heart failure Infective endocarditis Pulmonary hypertension

	ECHO: confirms diagnosis; allows severity to be assessed		Medical: manage heart failure and AF by following NICE guidelines		
			Surgical: valve repair is preferred since valve replacement may interfere with the function of the papillary muscles		

Table 1.2 Mitral Valve Disease

What is hypertension?
This is a clinic blood pressure that is >140/90 mmHg.

Pathophysiology
There is much uncertainty as to the cause of hypertension but it is likely multifactorial; ~95% of cases have no known cause and, in these cases, patients are said to have 'essential hypertension'.

More rarely, patients will have secondary hypertension. This should be considered in young patients with an acute onset of hypertension, any history that is suggestive of a renal or endocrine cause and when the patient fails to respond to medical therapy. Examples include renovascular disease, Conn's syndrome, Cushing's disease and phaeochromocytoma.

Blood pressure is controlled by several mechanisms, e.g. the autonomic nervous system, the capillary fluid shift mechanism, the renin–angiotensin–aldosterone system and adrenaline. A problem with one of these mechanisms may result in high blood pressure.

Lifestyle factors such as smoking, alcohol intake, obesity and stress also play a role in increasing blood pressure.

Investigations
- Clinic blood pressure readings (with ambulatory blood pressure monitoring to confirm). Stages of hypertension are listed below:

Blood pressure (mmHg)	Systolic	Diastolic
Normal	<120	<80
Pre-hypertension	120–139	80–89
Stage 1	140–159	90–99
Stage 2	160–179	100–109
Severe hypertension	≥180	≥110

- Bloods: FBC, LFTs, U&Es, creatinine, serum urea, eGFR, lipid levels and glucose.
- ECG: left ventricular hypertrophy.
- Urine dipstick: haematuria and proteinuria.

MAP 1.6 **Hypertension**

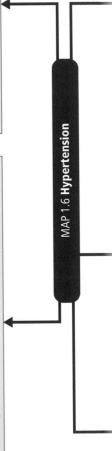

Causes

- Unknown: 'essential hypertension'.
- Secondary causes: renal and endocrine disease.
- Contributory lifestyle factors such as increased stress, smoking and obesity.

Complications

- MI.
- Heart failure.
- Renal impairment.
- Stroke.
- Hypertensive retinopathy.

Treatment

- Conservative: lifestyle advice including smoking cessation, encouraging weight loss, decreased alcohol consumption and a salt-restricted diet. Calculate 10-year risk of cardiovascular risk, e.g. QRisk score.
- Medical: this is split into 4 steps according to NICE guidelines:

	<55 years old or hyper-tension with diabetes		>55 years old or black-African/African–Caribbean patients or patients without diabetes	
Step 1	A		C	or D
Step 2	A + C	or	A + C	or A + D
Step 3	A + C + D			
Step 4	Refer for add-on therapy			

Key:
A: angiotensin converting enzyme (ACE) inhibitor or angiotensin receptor blocker (ARB) if ACE inhibitor is not tolerated by patient;
C: calcium channel blocker;
D: thiazide-type diuretic;
add-on therapy: spironolactone (side effect: hyperkalaemia), alpha-blocker or beta-blocker.

- Surgical: surgical excision (if related to cause).

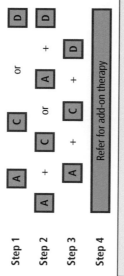

FIGURE 1.2 The Renin–Angiotensin System

Renin

Angiotensinogen → Angiotensin I → Angiotensin II

Angiotensin converting enzyme (ACE)

Angiotensin II stimulates:
- Aldosterone secretion from the zona glomerulosa of the adrenal cortex.
- Vasoconstriction.
- Antidiuretic hormone (ADH) release from the posterior pituitary gland.
- The sympathetic system.

Map 1.6 Hypertension

Map 1.7 Atrial Fibrillation (AF)

What is AF?

This is the most common tachyarrhythmia, characterised by an irregularly irregular pulse, rapid heart rate and ECG changes.

Signs and symptoms

- None.
- Palpitations.
- Dyspnoea.
- Syncope.
- Exercise intolerance.
- Fatigue.
- Heart failure.
- Irregularly irregular pulse.

Pathophysiology

Atrial ectopic beats, thought to originate in the pulmonary veins, lead to dysfunction of the cardiac electrical signalling pathway. As a result the atria no longer contract in a coordinated manner. Instead they fibrillate and contract irregularly. Due to the irregular contractions, the atria fail to empty adequately. This may result in stagnant blood accumulating within the atrial appendage, increasing the risk of clot formation and therefore embolic stroke.

Investigations

- Bloods: looking for reversible causes – FBC, U&E, LFTs, CRP, TFTs, calcium, phosphate, magnesium, HbA1c, cholesterol, septic screen (if applicable).
- Scoring systems: CHA2DS2-VASc stroke risk score, ORBIT bleeding risk score.
- Assessment of cardiac function: ECG (absent p waves, irregular RR intervals, undulating baseline, narrow QRS complexes), ambulatory 24-hour ECG monitoring, ECHO to assess valves or regional wall motion abnormalities.

MAP 1.7 **Atrial Fibrillation (AF)**

Causes

- Idiopathic.
- Ischaemic heart disease.
- Heart failure.
- Valve disease: mitral stenosis and mitral regurgitation.
- Hypertension.
- Hyperthyroidism.
- Alcohol induced.
- Familial.

Complications

- Stroke.
- Heart failure.
- Sudden death.

Treatment

Treatment varies depending on whether this is in the acute or non-acute setting.

- Acute setting:
  - Patients with life-threatening haemodynamic instability caused by AF may require electrical cardioversion. Always seek senior support.
  - Acutely but without haemodynamic instability requires rate and/or rhythm control. In the presence of concurrent heart failure seek further medical support.
- Non-acute setting:
  - Conservative: patient education, assessment and management of cardiovascular risk factors, e.g. smoking cessation, weight loss, decreasing alcohol intake.
  - Medical: correction of underlying cause, e.g. hyperthyroidism.
    - Rate control: beta-blocker, calcium channel blocker as initial monotherapy. Digoxin may be considered: 1. if the patient does no or very little physical exercise; 2. other rate-limiting drug options are ruled out because of comorbidities or the person's preferences.
    - If this does not work, combination therapy may be considered with a beta-blocker/diltiazem/digoxin.
    - Rhythm restoration: options include 1. cardioversion, e.g. with amiodarone or 2. long-term control, e.g. with a beta-blocker.
    - Stroke prevention – anticoagulants, e.g. warfarin, apixaban, rivaroxaban.
  - Surgery: pacing and atrioventricular node ablation if with permanent AF and symptoms or left ventricular dysfunction thought to be caused by high ventricular rates.

Map 1.7 Atrial Fibrillation (AF)

Figure 2.1 Respiratory Function Tests

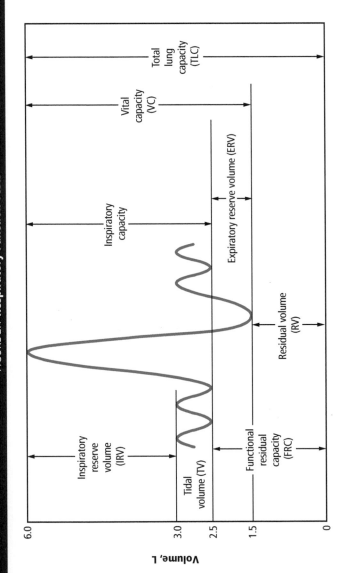

FIGURE 2.1 **Respiratory Function Tests**

TLC = VC + RV.

TLC = TV + RV + IRV + ERV.

VC = maximal exhalation after maximal inhalation.

RV = lung volume after maximal exhalation.

TV = volume of air with normal inhalation and exhalation.

FRC = ERV + RV. This is the lung volume after normal exhalation. It is decreased with atelectasis, sepsis (ARDS) and trauma.

ERV = the volume of air that can be forcefully expired after normal expiration.

FEV_1 = forced expiratory volume in 1 second.

Dead space = the area of the lung that is ventilated but not perfused. This is increased with pulmonary embolism, pulmonary hypertension and ARDS.

Ageing decreases FEV_1 and VC but increases FRC.

Ventilation/perfusion mismatch is greatest in the upper lobes of the lung.

Compliance = change in volume/change in pressure.

Patterns in restrictive lung disease = FEV_1 is normal or increased. TLC, RV and FVC are decreased.

Patterns in obstructive lung disease = FVC is normal or decreased. FEV_1 is decreased. TLC and RV are increased.

Figure 2.1 Respiratory Function Tests

Pathophysiology

- Chronic bronchitis: chronic infection results in the chronic infiltration of the respiratory submucosa by inflammatory cells. This results in mucous gland hyperplasia and smooth muscle hypertrophy, causing bronchial lumen narrowing. 'Blue bloaters' are patients in whom this pathology dominates.

- Emphysema: alveolar walls are destroyed resulting in bullae formation and the fusion of adjacent alveoli. This ultimately results in a decreased surface area for gas exchange and decreased elastic recoil with subsequent air trapping. 'Pink puffers' are patients in whom this pathology dominates.

Causes

Remember this as **GASES**:

- **Genetics**: alpha-1 antitrypsin deficiency results in the loss of protection against proteases.
- **Air** pollution.
- **Smoking**.
- **Exposure** through occupation, e.g. coal mining.
- **Secondhand** smoke exposure.

What is COPD?

This is a chronic obstructive airway disease that is characterised by its irreversibility.
It is closely linked to smoking.
It is made up of:

- Chronic bronchitis: cough with sputum production for at least 3 months in 2 consecutive years.
- Emphysema: this encompasses permanently dilated airways distal to the terminal bronchioles with alveolar destruction and bullae formation. It is defined histologically and is associated with alpha-1 antitrypsin deficiency and increased elastase activity.

MAP 2.1 **Chronic Obstructive Pulmonary Disease (COPD)**

Investigations

- Diagnosis is confirmed by spirometry, which has a FEV_1 value <80% predicted and FEV_1/FVC <0.7.
- CXR shows lung hyperinflation, emphysematous change and diaphragmatic flattening.
- Bloods: FBC, U&Es, WCC, ESR, CRP, alpha-1 antitrypsin levels.
- ECG: for cor pulmonale.
- Sputum culture.

The **GOLD scale** assesses severity of COPD:

Stage I: mild COPD.

Stage II: moderate COPD.

Stage III: severe COPD.

Stage IV: very severe COPD.

Complications

Remember this as **CLIPPeR**:

- **C**or pulmonale: right-sided heart failure due to chronic pulmonary hypertension.
- **L**ung cancer.
- **I**nfections: usually treat with macrolide antibiotics.
- **P**neumothorax.
- **P**olycythaemia.
- **e**
- **R**espiratory failure.

Treatment

- Conservative: smoking cessation, influenza and pneumococcal vaccinations, pulmonary rehabilitation.
- Medical: antibiotics for infections (long-term azithromycin and erythromycin reduces exacerbations over 1 year), mucolytics/antioxidants, regular use of N-acetylcysteine and carbocysteine reduces the risk of exacerbations in select populations, oxygen therapy.
  - COPD inhaled therapies algorithm:
    - Step 1: SABA or SAMA.
    - Step 2: if there are no asthmatic features, then LABA + LAMA. If there are asthmatic features, then consider LABA + ICS.
    - Step 3: if there are no asthmatic features and daily symptoms that affect quality of life, then consider a 3-month trial of LABA, LAMA and ICS. If there is no improvement, then revert to LABA or LAMA. If the patient has 2 moderate exacerbations or 1 severe exacerbation within 1 year, then consider LABA, LAMA and ICS. If there are asthmatic features with daily symptoms affecting quality of life or 2 moderate exacerbations or 1 severe exacerbation within 1 year, then offer LABA, LAMA and ICS.
    - Step 4: refer to specialist.

Map 2.1 Chronic Obstructive Pulmonary Disease (COPD)

What is asthma?

Asthma is a **chronic, inflammatory** disease that is characterised by **reversible** airway obstruction.

Signs and symptoms

- Wheezing.
- Shortness of breath.
- Coughing.

Remember to ask if the patient has a history of atopy, e.g. hay fever and eczema.

Triggering factors include:
- Dust/pets/vapours.
- Emotion.
- Drugs, e.g. beta-blockers.

Investigations

- Peak expiratory flow rate: note diurnal variation.
- Sputum sample.
- ABG: in emergency.
- Spirometry: for obstructive defects.
- Bloods: increased IgE, FBC.
- CXR: pneumothorax, consolidation.

Pathophysiology

- Copious mucus secretion.
- Inflammation.
- Contraction of bronchial muscle.

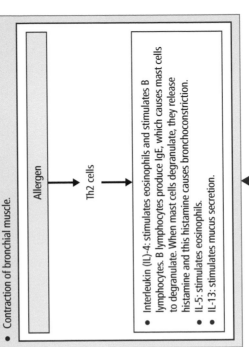

Allergen

↓

Th2 cells

↓

- Interleukin (IL)-4: stimulates eosinophils and stimulates B lymphocytes. B lymphocytes produce IgE, which causes mast cells to degranulate. When mast cells degranulate, they release histamine and this histamine causes bronchoconstriction.
- IL-5: stimulates eosinophils.
- IL-13: stimulates mucus secretion.

MAP 2.2 Asthma

Treatment

- Conservative: patient education; advice on inhaler technique and avoidance of triggering factors; annual asthma review and influenza vaccine required.
- Medical: refer to British Thoracic Society Guidelines: (see Appendix Two)
  - Step 1: low dose ICS with salbutamol not salbutamol alone.
  - Step 2: LABA + ICS.
  - Step 3: increase to medium dose ICS or add in LTRA, e.g. montelukast – if not responding to LABA then stop.
  - Step 4: refer to specialist.

Treatment of acute asthma

Remember as **O SHIT**:
- **O**xygen.
- **S**albutamol.
- **H**ydrocortisone.
- **I**pratropium.
- **T**heophylline.

Complications

- Death.
- Disturbed sleep.
- Persistent cough.
- Side effects of steroids:
  - Weight gain.
  - Thinning of the skin.
  - Striae formation.
  - Cataracts.
  - Cushing's syndrome.

Map 2.2 Asthma

Table 2.1 Type 1 vs. Type 2 Respiratory Failure

TABLE 2.1 Type 1 vs. Type 2 Respiratory Failure

	Type 1: hypoventilation with V/Q mismatch 'Pink puffer' – thin and hyperinflated	Type 2: hypoventilation with or without V/Q mismatch 'Blue bloater' – strong build and wheezy
Cause	Pneumonia Pulmonary embolism Pulmonary oedema Fibrosing alveolitis	Chronic obstructive pulmonary disease (COPD) and asthma Cerebrovascular disease Opiate overdose Myasthenia gravis Motor neuron disease
Symptoms	Remember this as **ABCD**: **A**gitation **B**reathlessness **C**onfusion **D**rowsiness and fatigue	Remember this as **ABCD**: **A**gitation **B**reathlessness **C**onfusion **D**rowsiness and fatigue
Signs	Central cyanosis	Remember this as **ABC**: **A** flapping tremor **B**ounding pulse **C**yanosis
PaO$_2$	↓ (<8.0 kPa)	↓ (<8.0 kPa)
PaCO$_2$	Normal (~6.7 kPa)	↑ (>6.7 kPa)
Treatment	Oxygen replacement therapy Treatment of underlying cause	Noninvasive ventilation Treatment of underlying cause
Complications	Nosocomial infections, e.g. pneumonia Heart failure Arrhythmia Pericarditis	Nosocomial infections, e.g. pneumonia Heart failure Arrhythmia Pericarditis

What is pneumonia?

Pneumonia is inflammation of the lung parenchyma caused by a lower respiratory tract infection. It often occurs after a viral infection in the upper respiratory tract. It is uncertain how the bacteria reach the lower respiratory tract after attaching to disaccharide receptors on pharyngeal epithelial cells.

Pathophysiology

Debatable methods of invasion include:

- The inhibition of IgA.
- Pneumolysins, which inhibit ciliary beating.
- Damage of the epithelial cells by prior infection.
- Hijacking the platelet aggregating factor receptor pathway to reach the alveoli.

Symptoms

- Fever.
- Cough with purulent sputum.
- Dyspnoea.
- Pleuritic pain.

Signs

- Percussion: dull.
- Auscultation: crackles, bronchial breathing.
- Respiratory failure: cyanosis, tachypnoea.
- Septicaemia: rigors.

Causative organisms

Children	Community-acquired pneumonia	Hospital-acquired pneumonia	HIV patients or immunocompromised patients
Viruses	Streptococcus pneumoniae	Gram-negative bacteria	Pneumocystis jirovecii
Pneumococcus	Haemophilus influenzae	Staphylococcus aureus	Cytomegalovirus
Mycoplasma	Moraxella catarrhalis	Streptococcus pneumoniae	Adenovirus
	Chlamydia pneumoniae (A)	Anaerobes	Herpes simplex virus
	Mycoplasma pneumoniae (A)	Fungi	Mycobacterium tuberculosis
	Legionella pneumophila (A)	Legionella pneumophila	Bacterial infection, e.g. Staphylococcus aureus
	Viruses		

A = Atypical

MAP 2.3 **Pneumonia**

Continued overleaf

Map 2.3 Pneumonia

Map 2.3 Pneumonia

MAP 2.3 **Pneumonia** (*Continued*)

Treatment

Remember this as **BAPP:**

- **B**reathing: maintain oxygen saturation levels.
- **A**ntibiotics: treat the underlying cause (check hospital guidelines).
- **P**ain: give analgesics.
- **P**neumococcal vaccines for those at risk, e.g. diabetics, the immunosuppressed and those over 65 years old.

Complications

- Respiratory failure: by causing acute respiratory distress syndrome (ARDS).
- Septic shock: the causative agent enters the patient's bloodstream, releasing cytokines.
- Pleural effusion.
- Empyema.
- Lung abscess.
- Hypotension: sepsis or dehydration is usually the underlying cause.

Investigations

- CXR: look for infiltrates.
- Identify the causative organism by assessing a sputum sample.
- Monitor oxygen saturation.
- Bloods: look for raised WCC and raised inflammatory markers.
- Urinary antigen test: for pneumococcal or *Legionella* antigen.
- Arterial blood gas (ABG).

Assess **severity** using **CURB-65**

- **C**onfusion.
- **U**rea >7 mmol/L.
- **R**espiratory rate >30/min.
- **B**P <90/<60 mmHg.
- **>65** years old.

Each section of the CURB-65 is worth 1 point:

1 = Outpatient care.

2 = Admission.

>3 = Requires ICU admission.

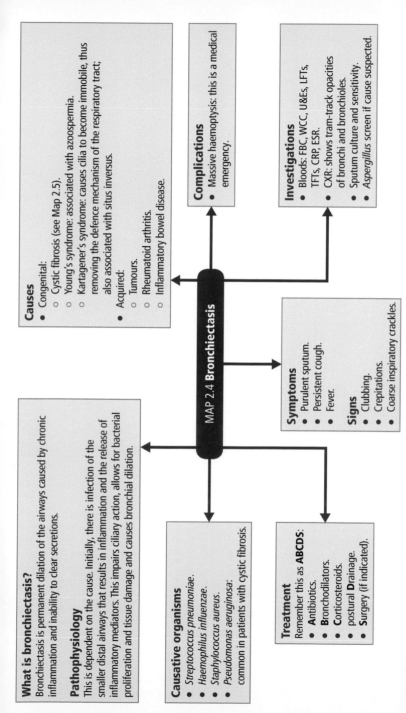

What is bronchiectasis?

Bronchiectasis is permanent dilation of the airways caused by chronic inflammation and inability to clear secretions.

Pathophysiology

This is dependent on the cause. Initially, there is infection of the smaller distal airways that results in inflammation and the release of inflammatory mediators. This impairs ciliary action, allows for bacterial proliferation and tissue damage and causes bronchial dilation.

Causative organisms

- *Streptococcus pneumoniae*.
- *Haemophilus influenzae*.
- *Staphylococcus aureus*.
- *Pseudomonas aeruginosa*: common in patients with cystic fibrosis.

Treatment

Remember this as **ABCDS**:
- **A**ntibiotics.
- **B**ronchodilators.
- **C**orticosteroids.
- postural **D**rainage.
- **S**urgery (if indicated).

MAP 2.4 Bronchiectasis

Causes

- Congenital:
  - Cystic fibrosis (see Map 2.5).
  - Young's syndrome: associated with azoospermia.
  - Kartagener's syndrome: causes cilia to become immobile, thus removing the defence mechanism of the respiratory tract; also associated with situs inversus.
- Acquired:
  - Tumours.
  - Rheumatoid arthritis.
  - Inflammatory bowel disease.

Complications

- Massive haemoptysis: this is a medical emergency.

Investigations

- Bloods: FBC, WCC, U&Es, LFTs, TFTs, CRP, ESR.
- CXR: shows tram-track opacities of bronchi and bronchioles.
- Sputum culture and sensitivity.
- *Aspergillus* screen if cause suspected.

Symptoms

- Purulent sputum.
- Persistent cough.
- Fever.

Signs

- Clubbing.
- Crepitations.
- Coarse inspiratory crackles.

Map 2.5 Cystic Fibrosis

What is cystic fibrosis?

Cystic fibrosis is a chronic disease that is inherited in an autosomal recessive pattern. It is a leading cause of bronchiectasis and it frequently leads to chronic sinopulmonary infections as well as pancreatic insufficiency.

Cause

- Mutation in a gene on chromosome 7 that codes for a protein transmembrane conductance regulator (CFTR) protein. This functions as a transmembrane cAMP-activated chloride channel.

Signs and symptoms

- Thickened mucus secretions of most organ systems resulting in plugging and obstruction pathologies – most frequently this includes the sinuses, the lungs, the hepatobiliary systems and the intestines.
- Meconium ileus.
- Chronic sinusitis (ciliary dysfunction and colonisation with *Pseudomonas aeruginosa* contributes to this).
- Malabsorption particularly of fat-soluble vitamins A, D, E and K due to thickened pancreatic secretions.
- Pancreatitis.
- Gallstones.
- Obstructive cirrhosis and post-hepatic hyperbilirubinemia can occur. Secondary to this, oesophageal varices, splenomegaly, and hypersplenism may occur as a result of increased hepatic portal vein pressures.
- Obstructive azoospermia.

Investigations

For a diagnostic pathway please see:
https://www.nice.org.uk/guidance/ng78/chapter/Recommendations#diagnosis-of-cystic-fibrosis
- Newborn screening panel
- Guthrie test in neonatal period which detects raised serum immunoreactive trypsinogen
- Evidence of CFTR dysfunction. Some tests that looks for CFTR dysfunction include:
  ○ Elevated sweat chloride >60 mmol/L on two occasions.
  ○ Two disease-causing *CFTR* mutations.
  ○ Abnormal nasal potential difference.
- Typically, the investigative pathway starts with sweat testing, if this is abnormal then DNA testing is indicated.
- Other investigations depend on symptoms and include things like blood tests looking for signs of infection, chest X-ray, etc.
- Bronchoalveolar lavage typically shows many neutrophils, and microbiology is commonly positive for *Haemophilus influenza*, *Staphylococcus aureus*, *Pseudomonas aeruginosa*, *Burkholderia cepacia*.
- Pulmonary function tests are useful to evaluate and monitor disease progression in CF.

MAP 2.5 **Cystic Fibrosis**

Treatment

- Conservative: MDT support, exercise, vitamin supplementation, DEXA scan, regular monitoring and pulmonary function tests, chest physiotherapy, fertility advice, try to keep cystic fibrosis sufferers separate in order to reduce cross infection.
- Medical: seek specialist input
  - Pulmonary management: airway clearance techniques, mucoactive agents, e.g. rhDNase, a recombinant human deoxyribonuclease is the first-line agent, consider mannitol dry powder for inhalation with specialist input.
  - Diagnose and treat pulmonary infection.
  - Patient with deteriorating lung function or repeated pulmonary exacerbations may be offered long-term treatment with an immuno-modulatory agent such as azithromycin.
  - Nutritional interventions and exocrine pancreatic insufficiency.
    - Dietician support regarding total nutritional intake, estimated nutritional needs and pancreatic enzyme replacement therapy, if appropriate.
  - Liver disease
    - Monitor liver function tests, if abnormal then an USS liver may be required.
    - Consider ursodeoxycholic acid treatment.
    - Refer people to a liver specialist if any of the following:
      - Chronic progressive liver disease.
      - Liver failure, based on clinical assessment and liver function tests.
      - Portal hypertension, haematemesis, splenomegaly or findings on liver ultrasound scan.
- Surgical: consider lung transplant in certain cases.

Complications

- Meconium ileus (affects 1 in 7 newborn babies).
- Fat-soluble vitamin deficiencies.
- Muscle pains and arthralgia.
- Male infertility caused by obstructive azoospermia.
- Reduced female fertility.
- Upper airway complications, including nasal polyps and sinusitis.
- Chronic liver disease.
- Gallstones and renal stones.
- Cystic-fibrosis-related diabetes (uncommon in children under 10 years, but the prevalence increases with age and it affects up to 1 in 2 adults).
- Osteoporosis.

Map 2.5 Cystic Fibrosis

Map 2.6 Pneumoconiosis

Berylliosis

- Caused by inhaling beryllium.
- It causes granuloma formation, made up of:
  - Giant cells.
  - Macrophages.
  - Epithelioid cells.

Other granulomatous conditions include: tuberculosis, leprosy, cat-scratch disease and sarcoidosis.

Silicosis

- This is also known as Potter's rot.
- Caused by inhaling silica particles, which cannot be removed by respiratory defences.
- Macrophages engulf the silica particles releasing tumour necrosis factor (TNF) and cytokines that induce fibroblasts, resulting in fibrosis and collagen deposition.
- Associated with increased tuberculosis (TB) infection.
- Eggshell calcification of hilar lymph nodes is apparent on CXR, along with nodular lesions in the upper lobes.

Bauxite fibrosis

- This is also known as Shaver's disease.
- Caused by inhaling bauxite fumes.

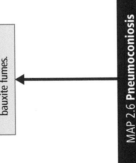

MAP 2.6 Pneumoconiosis

Siderosis

- Caused by inhaling iron particles.
- Benign with no apparent respiratory symptoms or altered lung function.

Coal workers' pneumoconiosis

- Caused by inhaling coal dust.
- The dust particles accumulate in the lung parenchyma and are engulfed by macrophages. These macrophages then die, releasing enzymes, resulting in tissue fibrosis.

Asbestosis

- Caused by inhaling asbestos fibres. The fusiform rods are found inside macrophages.
- Associated with malignant mesothelioma.
- Pleural plaques are apparent on CXR.
- White asbestos has the lowest fibrogenicity, whereas blue asbestos has the highest.

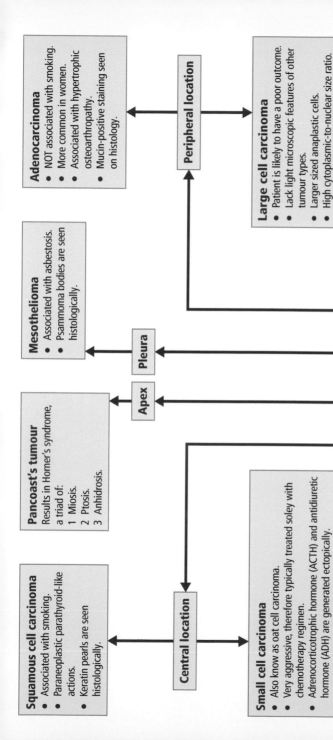

Adenocarcinoma
- NOT associated with smoking.
- More common in women.
- Associated with hypertrophic osteoarthropathy.
- Mucin-positive staining seen on histology.

Large cell carcinoma
- Patient is likely to have a poor outcome.
- Lack light microscopic features of other tumour types.
- Larger sized anaplastic cells.
- High cytoplasmic-to-nuclear size ratio.
- Treated by surgical excision of tumour.

Peripheral location

Mesothelioma
- Associated with asbestosis.
- Psammoma bodies are seen histologically.

Pancoast's tumour
Results in Horner's syndrome, a triad of:
1 Miosis.
2 Ptosis.
3 Anhidrosis.

Pleura

Apex

MAP 2.7 Lung Cancer

Central location

Squamous cell carcinoma
- Associated with smoking.
- Paraneoplastic parathyroid-like actions.
- Keratin pearls are seen histologically.

Small cell carcinoma
- Also know as oat cell carcinoma.
- Very aggressive, therefore typically treated soley with chemotherapy regimen.
- Adrenocorticotrophic hormone (ACTH) and antidiuretic hormone (ADH) are generated ectopically.
- Associated with Lambert–Eaton syndrome.
- Kulchitsky cells are seen histologically.
- Non-small cell carcinomas (NSCCs) are any epithelial derived lung cancers that are not small cell carcinoma (SCC). They are relatively insensitive to chemotherapy.

Continued overleaf

Map 2.7 Lung Cancer

Map 2.7 Lung Cancer

MAP 2.7 **Lung Cancer** (*Continued*)

What is lung cancer?
- 2nd commonest cancer in the UK.
- Onset age 60–80 years and more common in males.
- Many different types and may be characterised as central or peripheral (as described above).

Risk factors
- Smoking.
- Occupational exposure, e.g. asbestos (blue asbestos has maximum fibrogenicity).

Symptoms
- Cough.
- Dyspnoea.
- Haemoptysis.
- Chest wall/bone pain.
- Weight loss.
- Fatigue.
- Neuro symptoms.

Signs
- Weight loss.
- Clubbing.
- Use of accessory muscles.
- Dull to percussion (pleural effusion).

Investigations
- Bloods: FBC, U&E (SIADH in small cell), calcium, LDH (bone mets), LFTs (mets).
- Radiology: chest X-ray.
- CT chest and complete staging CT, flexible bronchoscopy +/– FNA.
- MRI brain.

Treatment
Conservative, medical or surgical depending on the type of cancer, the stage and the grade. Requires MDT input.

Differential diagnosis
of solitary pulmonary nodule includes:
- Lung cancer.
- Hamartoma.
- Granuloma.
- TB.
- Fungal infection.

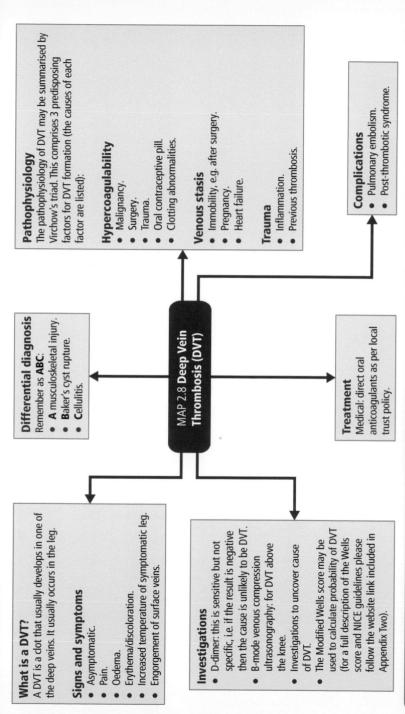

What is a DVT?

A DVT is a clot that usually develops in one of the deep veins. It usually occurs in the leg.

Signs and symptoms

- Asymptomatic.
- Pain.
- Oedema.
- Erythema/discoloration.
- Increased temperature of symptomatic leg.
- Engorgement of surface veins.

Investigations

- D-dimer: this is sensitive but not specific, i.e. if the result is negative then the cause is unlikely to be DVT.
- B-mode venous compression ultrasonography: for DVT above the knee.
- Investigations to uncover cause of DVT.
- The Modified Wells score may be used to calculate probability of DVT (for a full description of the Wells score and NICE guidelines please follow the website link included in Appendix Two).

Differential diagnosis

Remember as **ABC**:

- **A** musculoskeletal injury.
- **B**aker's cyst rupture.
- **C**ellulitis.

MAP 2.8 Deep Vein Thrombosis (DVT)

Pathophysiology

The pathophysiology of DVT may be summarised by Virchow's triad. This comprises 3 predisposing factors for DVT formation (the causes of each factor are listed):

Hypercoagulability

- Malignancy.
- Surgery.
- Trauma.
- Oral contraceptive pill.
- Clotting abnormalities.

Venous stasis

- Immobility, e.g. after surgery.
- Pregnancy.
- Heart failure.

Trauma

- Inflammation.
- Previous thrombosis.

Complications

- Pulmonary embolism.
- Post-thrombotic syndrome.

Treatment

Medical: direct oral anticoagulants as per local trust policy.

Map 2.8 Deep Vein Thrombosis (DVT)

Map 2.9 Pulmonary Embolism (PE)

MAP 2.9 Pulmonary Embolism (PE)

What is a PE?

This is occlusion of the pulmonary vasculature by a clot. Often it occurs from a deep vein thrombosis (DVT) that has become dislodged and forms an embolus that lodges in the pulmonary arterial vasculature, blocking the vessels.

Signs and symptoms

- Breathlessness: this may be of sudden onset or progressive.
- Tachypnoea.
- Pleuritic chest pain.
- Tachycardia.
- Cyanosis.
- Haemoptysis.
- Palpitations.

Causes

- DVT.
- Air embolus.
- Fat embolus.
- Amniotic fluid embolus.
- Foreign material introduced via IV drug use.

Pathophysiology

The extent of thrombus may be classified into small–medium, multiple and massive PE. Symptom correlation depends on where the pulmonary circulation is occluded.

There are 3 pathways involved in the pathophysiology of PE:

1. Platelet factor release: serotonin and thromboxane A_2 cause vasoconstriction.
2. Decreased alveolar perfusion: lung is underperfused and this leads to diminished gas exchange.
3. Decreased surfactant: this leads to ventilation/perfusion mismatch, hypoxaemia and dyspnoea.

Complications

- Sudden death.
- Arrhythmia.
- Pulmonary infarction.
- Pleural effusion.
- Paradoxical embolism.
- Pulmonary hypertension.

Treatment

- Acute:
  - Oxygen.
  - IV fluids.
  - Thrombolysis therapy if indicated, e.g. alteplase if massive PE or haemodynamically unstable.
  - Low molecular weight heparin.
- Long-term management:
  - Anticoagulation.
  - Inferior vena cava filter.

Investigations

- D-dimer: sensitive but not specific; negative result used to rule out PE.
- Thrombophilia screening: in patients <50 years with recurrent PE.
- CXR: usually normal.
- ECG: sinus tachycardia, S1Q3T3 pattern is classical but rare; excludes MI.
- ABG: hypoxaemia.
- CT, pulmonary angiography.
- V/Q scan.
- The Wells score may be used to calculate risk of PE. The factors may be found at: https://www.mdcalc.com/wells-criteria-pulmonary-embolism

Pathophysiology

The pathophysiology of pneumothorax is directly linked to cause, outlined below.

- Primary spontaneous pneumothorax:
  - Idiopathic/rupture of pleural bleb.
  - Usually found in young, tall, slim men.
- Secondary spontaneous pneumothorax:
  - In patients with prior lung disease, e.g. COPD, sarcoidosis or idiopathic pulmonary fibrosis.
- Tension pneumothorax:
  - Due to blunt, traumatic injuries, e.g. a stab wound.
  - Air cannot be removed on expiration due to one-way valve mechanism. This leads to mediastinal shift and lung collapse.

Complications

- Risk of future pneumothorax.
- Respiratory failure.
- Cardiac arrest.

Causes

- Ruptured pleural bleb.
- Chronic obstructive pulmonary disease (COPD).
- Tuberculosis.
- Sarcoidosis.
- Idiopathic pulmonary fibrosis.
- Rheumatoid arthritis.
- Ankylosing spondylitis.
- Lung cancer.
- Trauma, e.g. stab wound.

MAP 2.10 Pneumothorax

Treatment

- If pneumothorax on CXR <2 cm then no treatment is required; advise patients not to travel by air or to dive.
- If >2 cm then aspirate air +/– intercostal drain.
- Tension pneumothorax requires immediate decompression with a large-bore needle inserted into the 2nd intercostal space mid-clavicular line.

What is a pneumothorax?

A pneumothorax is air within the pleural space.

Signs and symptoms

- Ipsilateral chest pain.
- Shoulder tip pain.
- Dyspnoea.
- Tachypnoea.
- Hypoxia.
- Cyanosis.
- Auscultation: decreased on affected side.
- Percussion: hyper-resonant or normal.

Investigations

- CXR: pleural line; may show tracheal deviation away from lesion.
- CT scan +/– trauma series.
- ABG: hypoxia.

Map 2.10 Pneumothorax

FIGURE 3.1 **Causes of Regional Abdominal Pain**

Right hypochondriac region
- Pancreatitis
- Ulcer (gastric)
- Gallstones
- Biliary colic

Epigastric region
- Heartburn
- Pancreatitis
- Epigastric hernia
- Gallstones
- Ulcer (gastric)

Left hypochondriac region
- Pancreatitis
- Ulcer (gastric or duodenal)

Right lumbar region
- Kidney stones
- Urinary tract infection
- Constipation

Umbilical region
- Gastric ulcer
- Early stages of appendicitis
- Aortic aneurysm
- Ruptured aortic aneurysm
- Pancreatitis
- IBD

Left lumbar region
- Kidney stones
- Urinary tract infection
- Constipation
- Diverticular disease

Right iliac region
- Appendicitis
- Ectopic pregnancy
- Ovarian torsion
- Inguinal or femoral hernias
- Inflammatory bowel disease (IBD)

Hypogastric region
- Urinary tract infection
- Appendicitis
- IBD
- Diverticular disease

Left iliac region
- Diverticular disease
- IBD
- Ectopic pregnancy
- Ovarian torsion
- Inguinal or femoral hernias

Figure 3.1 Causes of Regional Abdominal Pain

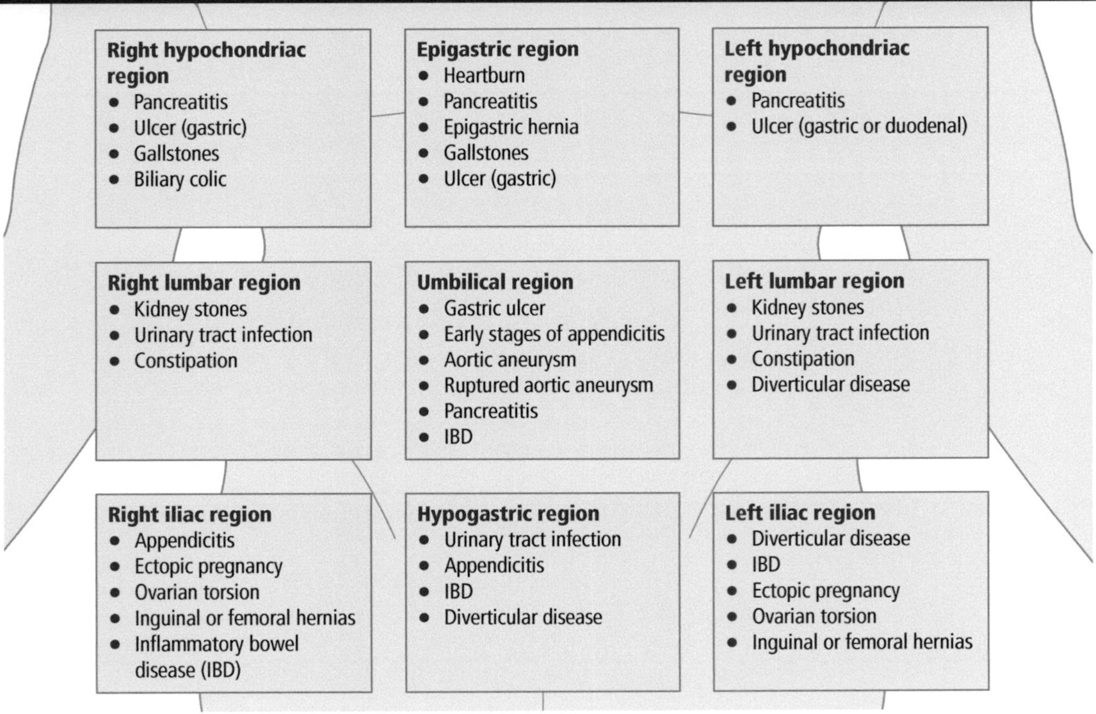

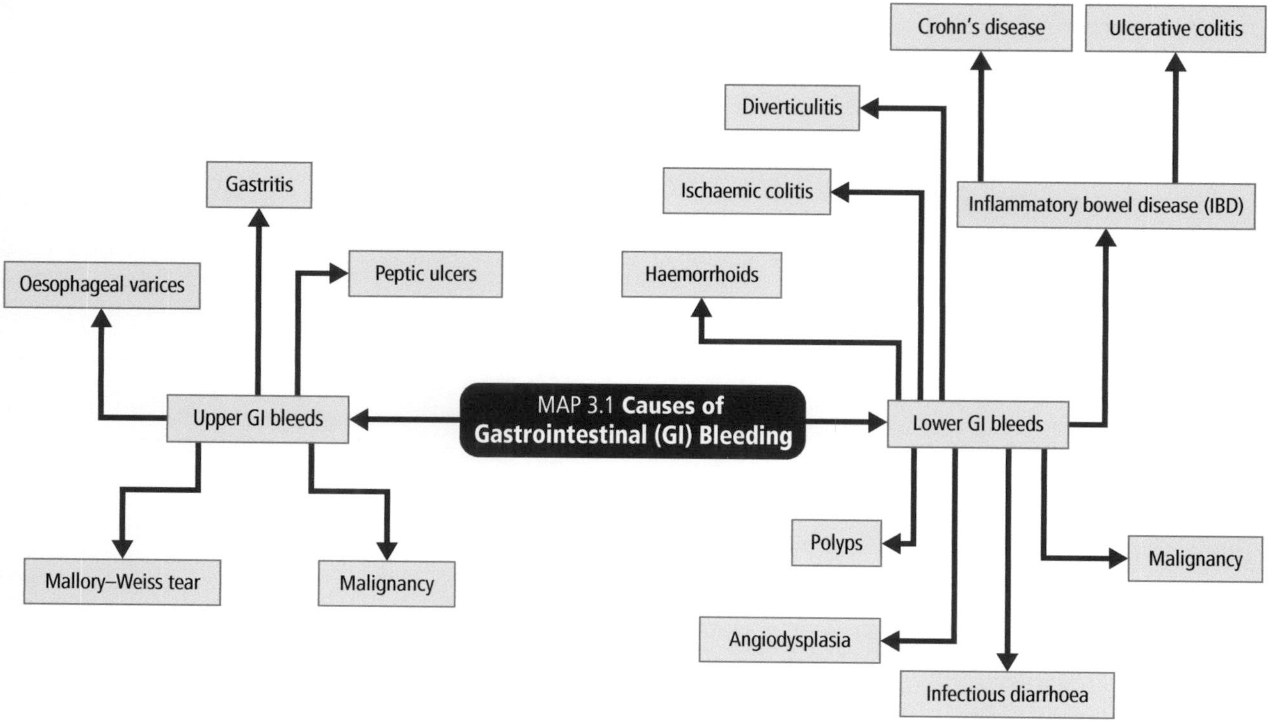
MAP 3.1 Causes of Gastrointestinal (GI) Bleeding
Upper GI bleeds
Oesophageal varices
Gastritis
Peptic ulcers
Mallory–Weiss tear
Malignancy
Lower GI bleeds
Haemorrhoids
Ischaemic colitis
Diverticulitis
Crohn's disease
Ulcerative colitis
Inflammatory bowel disease (IBD)
Polyps
Angiodysplasia
Infectious diarrhoea
Malignancy

GASTRITIS

What is gastritis?

This is inflammation of the stomach lining. Gastritis may be acute or chronic.

- Acute gastritis, caused by:
  - ○ Stress.
  - ○ NSAIDs.
  - ○ Uraemia.
  - ○ Burns: Curling's ulcer.
  - ○ Alcohol.

- Chronic gastritis:
  - ○ Type A:
    - – Autoimmune: autoantibodies are present to parietal cells.
    - – Presents with pernicious anaemia.
    - – Occurs in the fundus or body of the stomach.
  - ○ Type B:
    - – Most common.
    - – Associated with *Helicobacter pylori* infection.

Investigate for *H. pylori* infection

H. pylori is a Gram-negative, micro-aerophilic, spiral bacterium. It can form biofilms and produces urease, oxidase and catalase.

- Bloods: anaemia and *H. pylori*.
- Urinalysis.
- Blood test – measures antibodies to *H. pylori*.
- Carbon isotope–urea breath test.
- Endoscopy with biopsy of stomach lining.
- Stool microscopy and culture – may detect trace amounts of *H. pylori*.

Treatment

- Triple therapy to eradicate *H. pylori*: proton pump inhibitor (PPI), with amoxicillin 1 g and clarithromycin 500 mg or metronidazole 400 mg and clarithromycin 250 mg, taken twice daily.
- Step-wise approach to treating gastritis:
  - ○ Mild – antacids or H_2-receptor antagonists. N.B. Ranitidine is no longer prescribed due to the increased risk of ductal carcinoma.
  - ○ Moderate/severe – PPI. Side effects of PPI include increased risk of *Clostridium difficile*, low magnesium, pneumonia, and increased risk of hip, spine and wrist fractures.

Complications

- Peptic ulcers, anaemia (from bleeding ulcers), stricture formation, mucosa-associated lymphoid tissue (MALT) lymphoma.

IRRITABLE BOWEL SYNDROME (IBS)

What is IBS?

This is a common functional disorder of the bowel.

Signs and symptoms

Recurrent abdominal pain, which improves with defecation; there is a change in bowel habit, i.e. increased or decreased frequency.

Investigations

This is a clinical diagnosis.

Treatment

- Conservative: education and avoidance of triggering factors, e.g. decrease stress.
- Medical: depends on symptoms; antimuscarinics, laxatives, stool softeners, antispasmodics and antidepressants may play a role.

Complications

- Depression and anxiety.

APPENDICITIS

What is appendicitis?

This is inflammation of the appendix that presents with pain that can originate in the umbilical area before migrating to the right iliac fossa.

Investigations

Diagnosis is clinical:

- Bloods: FBC, U&Es, CRP.
- Ultrasound.
- Pregnancy test in females of child-bearing age to rule out ectopic pregnancy. CT scan in >50 year olds (follow trust guidelines) to exclude caecal tumour.
- Alvarado Score for Acute Appendicitis: A score of 5 or 6 is compatible with the diagnosis of acute appendicitis, a score of 7 or 8 indicates a probable appendicitis, a score of 9 or 10 indicates a very probable appendicitis.

The components comprising this score include right lower quadrant tenderness, elevated temperature, rebound tenderness, migration of pain to the right iliac fossa, anorexia, nausea and vomiting, leukocytosis and leucocyte left shift. The scoring system may be found here: https://www.mdcalc.com/alvarado-score-acute-appendicitis

Treatment

- Medical: analgesia and antibiotics as per local trust policy. Sometimes patients are treated solely using this method depending on risk factors, e.g. multiple comorbidities + COVID-19. Consultant surgeon decision.
- Surgical: laparoscopic or open appendicectomy.

Complications

- Peritonitis.
- Abscess formation.
- Death.
- Sepsis.
- Appendix mass.
- Incidental finding of carcinoid tumour requiring further surgical intervention (right hemi-colectomy).

MAP 3.2 **Causes of Gastrointestinal (GI) Inflammation**

Inflammatory bowel disease (IBD)

Continued overleaf

Map 3.2 Causes of Gastrointestinal (GI) Inflammation

Inflammatory bowel disease (IBD) (Continued)

CROHN'S DISEASE

What is Crohn's disease?

This is a disordered response to intestinal bacteria with transmural inflammation. It may affect any part of the gastrointestinal tract but often targets the terminal ileum. It is associated with granuloma formation.

Signs and symptoms

- Weight loss, abdominal pain (with palpable mass), diarrhoea, fever, skip lesions, clubbing, cobblestone mucosa, fistula formation, fissure formation and linear ulceration.

Investigations

- Bloods: FBC and platelets, U&Es, LFTs and albumin, ESR and CRP. Faecal calprotectin.
- Colonoscopy (with biopsy): diagnostic.
- Radiology: small bowel follow-through (diagnostic) and abdominal X-ray (for toxic megacolon and excluding perforation).

Treatment

- Conservative: smoking cessation, low residue diet may be encouraged but usually diet is normal.
- Medical: corticosteroids, infliximab, 5-ASA analogues (sulfasalazine), azathioprine, methotrexate.
- Surgical: remove strictured or obstructed region of bowel.

Complications

- Stricture formation, fistula formation, obstruction, pyoderma gangrenosum, anaemia and osteoporosis.

ULCERATIVE COLITIS

What is ulcerative colitis?

This is a relapsing remitting autoimmune condition that is not associated with granulomas. It affects the colon and rarely the terminal ileum (backwash ileitis).

Signs and symptoms

Remember the **5Ps**:

- **P**yrexia.
- **P**seudopolyps.
- lead **P**ipe radiological appearances.
- **P**oo (bloody diarrhoea).
- **P**roctitis.

Investigations

- These are the same as Crohn's disease.

Treatment

- Conservative: patient education; smoking has been shown to be protective but is not advised.
- Medical: corticosteroids, 5-aminosalicylic acid (5-ASA) analogues (sulfasalazine), mesalazine, 6-mercaptopurine, azathioprine.
- Surgical: colectomy.

Complications

- Toxic megacolon, increased incidence of colon cancer, primary sclerosing cholangitis and osteoporosis (from steroid use).

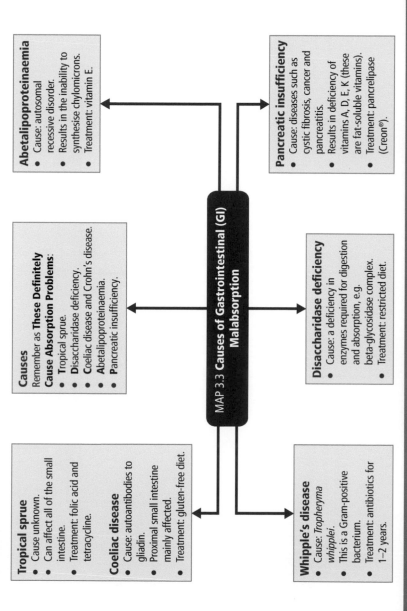

Abetalipoproteinaemia
- Cause: autosomal recessive disorder.
- Results in the inability to synthesise chylomicrons.
- Treatment: vitamin E.

Causes
Remember as **These Definitely Cause Absorption Problems**:
- **T**ropical sprue.
- **D**isaccharidase deficiency.
- **C**oeliac disease and Crohn's disease.
- **A**betalipoproteinaemia.
- **P**ancreatic insufficiency.

MAP 3.3 **Causes of Gastrointestinal (GI) Malabsorption**

Tropical sprue
- Cause unknown.
- Can affect all of the small intestine.
- Treatment: folic acid and tetracycline.

Coeliac disease
- Cause: autoantibodies to gliadin.
- Proximal small intestine mainly affected.
- Treatment: gluten-free diet.

Whipple's disease
- Cause: *Tropheryma whipplei*.
- This is a Gram-positive bacterium.
- Treatment: antibiotics for 1–2 years.

Disaccharidase deficiency
- Cause: a deficiency in enzymes required for digestion and absorption, e.g. beta-glycosidase complex.
- Treatment: restricted diet.

Pancreatic insufficiency
- Cause: diseases such as cystic fibrosis, cancer and pancreatitis.
- Results in deficiency of vitamins A, D, E, K (these are fat-soluble vitamins).
- Treatment: pancrelipase (Creon®).

Map 3.3 Causes of Gastrointestinal (GI) Malabsorption

Map 3.4 Gastro-oesophageal Reflux Disease (GORD)

Investigations

Age dependent:
- If the patient is <55 years old:
  ○ Proceed to treatment unless they have ALARM symptoms, e.g. unintentional weight loss, dysphagia, haematemesis, melaena and anorexia.
- If >55 years old:
  ○ Send patient to endoscopy: diagnostic and allows for biopsy.
  ○ 24-h pH monitoring.

Causes

- Genetic inheritance of angle of lower oesophageal sphincter.
- Oesophagitis.
- Sliding hiatus hernia.
- Rolling hiatus hernia.

Risk factors

- Smoking.
- Excessive alcohol.
- Excessive coffee.
- Obesity.
- Pregnancy.
- Drugs, e.g. calcium channel blockers, antimuscarinics and tricyclic antidepressants.

What is GORD?

This is abnormal reflux where acid from the stomach refluxes into the oesophagus, subsequently damaging the squamous oesophageal lining, causing discomfort.

Signs and symptoms

- Heartburn – pain is worse in certain positions, e.g. lying down/stooping and is worse after heavy meals.
- Regurgitation.
  ○ Water brash (excess salivation).
- Dysphagia.
- Nocturnal asthma/chronic cough.
- Laryngitis.

MAP 3.4 Gastro-oesophageal Reflux Disease (GORD)

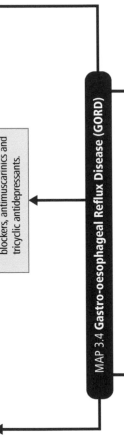

Treatment

- Conservative: education, weight loss, raising head of bed at night and avoidance of precipitating factors, e.g. smoking, large meals.
- Medical:
  - Antacids, e.g. aluminium hydroxide.
  - H_2-receptor antagonists, e.g. cimetidine.
  - Proton pump inhibitors, e.g. omeprazole.
- Surgical: Nissen's fundoplication.

Complications: Barrett's oesophagus

What is Barrett's oesophagus?

This is metaplasia of the normal squamous epithelium of the lower oesophagus to columnar epithelium. This occurs in patients who suffer with GORD for several years.

It is a premalignant lesion.

Investigations

- Endoscopy with biopsy in all 4 quadrants.

Treatment

- HALO® system radiofrequency ablation or mucosal resection for highly dysplastic lesions.

Complications

- Adenocarcinoma of the oesophagus.

Map 3.4 Gastro-oesophageal Reflux Disease (GORD)

Map 3.5 Jaundice

What is jaundice?

Jaundice, also known as icterus, is the yellow discoloration of mucous membranes, sclera and skin.

This happens due to the accumulation of bilirubin. Jaundice may be seen at a bilirubin concentration >2.5–3.0 mg/dL (42.8–51.3 mmol/L).

Causes

The causes of jaundice may be split into 3 categories (see table below):

1 Prehepatic jaundice.
2 Intrahepatic jaundice.
3 Posthepatic jaundice.

Treatment

Treat the underlying cause.

Complications

- Liver failure.
- Renal failure.
- Sepsis.
- Pancreatitis.
- Biliary cirrhosis.
- Cholangitis.
- Kernicterus (a serious complication of jaundice in neonates).

Investigations

You must determine underlying cause.
Use these tests to determine the type of jaundice:

- Appearance of urine and stool.
- LFTs.
- Bilirubin levels.
- Alkaline phosphatase levels.
- Gamma-glutamyl transferase.
- Coagulation profile (PT best marker of liver synthetic function).
- U&E.
- Non-invasive liver screen.
- Hepatitis serology +/– HIV in at-risk individuals.
- Radiology: USS liver and biliary tree, MRCP +/– ERCP.

The different blood results for different types of jaundice:

Investigations	Prehepatic jaundice	Intrahepatic jaundice	Posthepatic jaundice
Appearance of urine	Normal	Dark	Dark
Appearance of stool	Normal	Pale	Pale
Conjugated bilirubin	Normal	↑	↑
Unconjugated bilirubin	Normal or ↑	↑	Normal
Total bilirubin	Normal or ↑	↑	↑
Alkaline phosphatase	Normal	↑	↑

MAP 3.5 **Jaundice**

The causes of different types of jaundice

Prehepatic jaundice	Intrahepatic jaundice	Posthepatic jaundice
Crigler–Najjar syndrome	Viral hepatitis	Intraluminal – gallstones in the common bile duct
Gilbert's syndrome	Alcoholic liver disease	Mural causes – strictures, cholangiocarcinoma
Haemolytic causes, e.g. thalassaemia, sickle cell disease	Hepatocellular carcinoma	Extraluminal causes – Mirizzi's syndrome, pancreatic tumours
	Primary biliary cirrhosis	
	Primary sclerosis cholangitis	
	Autoimmune hepatitis	
	Hereditary haemochromatosis	
	Iatrogenic, i.e. drugs	

Map 3.6 Hepatitis Virus

HEPATITIS A (HAV)

What is HAV?

It is a RNA picornavirus.

Transmission

Faecal–oral transmission, associated with contaminated shellfish. The virus passes into bile after replication within liver cells. The immune system is activated by this process and leads to necrosis predominantly in zone 3 of the hepatic lobule.

Incubation period

• 2–3 weeks.

Investigations

• Anti-HAV IgM in serum.

Treatment

• Conservative: vaccine for travellers to endemic areas.
• Medical: supportive since HAV is often self-resolving.

Complications

• Rarely acute liver failure.

HEPATITIS B (HBV)

What is HBV?

A partially stranded, enveloped DNA virus. It has an e-antigen that indicates increased infectivity.

Transmission

• Vertical transmission.
• Contaminated needles.
• Infected blood products.
• Sexual intercourse.

Incubation period

• 1–5 months.

Investigations

HBV DNA in serum, HBsAg, HBeAg, anti-HBc; HBsAg presents on histology with a 'ground glass' appearance.

Treatment

• Conservative: education and prevention of disease; vaccine for at-risk groups, e.g. health workers.
• Medical: antiviral medications, e.g. pegylated interferon alpha-2a, adefovir, entecavir, lamivudine, tenofovir, telbivudine.

Complications

• Hepatic cirrhosis, hepatocellular carcinoma (HCC), fulminant hepatitis B.

MAP 3.6 **Hepatitis Virus**

HEPATITIS C (HCV)

What is HCV?
It is a single stranded, enveloped RNA virus and a member of the flavivirus family.

Transmission
- Vertical transmission (occasionally).
- Contaminated needles.
- Infected blood products.

Incubation period
- Intermediate (6–9 weeks).

Investigations
- Antibody to HCV in the serum.

Treatment
- Conservative: education and prevention of disease.
- Medical: antiviral medications, e.g. peglylated interferon alpha-2a, ribavirin, taribavirin, telaprevir.

Complications
- Hepatic cirrhosis, HCC, liver failure.

HEPATITIS D (HDV)

What is HDV?
It is a single stranded defective RNA virus that co-infects with hepatitis B virus. Co-infectivity with HDV leads to an increased chance of liver failure.

Transmission
- Contaminated needles.
- Infected blood products.
- Sexual intercourse (rare).

Incubation period
- 1–5 months.

Investigations
- Serum IgM anti-D.

Treatment
- Peglylated interferon alpha-2a.

Complications
- Hepatic cirrhosis, HCC.

HEPATITIS E (HEV)

What is HEV?
It is a single stranded RNA virus.

Transmission
- Faecal–oral transmission, associated with contaminated water.

Incubation period
- 2–3 weeks.

Investigations
- IgG and IgM anti-HEV.

Treatment
- Usually self-limiting.

Complications
- High mortality rate in pregnant women (~20%).

Map 3.6 Hepatitis Virus

Map 3.7 Colorectal Cancer (CRC)

What is CRC?

This is cancer of the colon and rectum and is the third most common malignancy. Usually adenocarcinoma on histology.

Signs and symptoms

- Abdominal pain.
- Unintentional weight loss.
- Altered bowel habit.
- Faecal occult blood.
- Anaemia.
- Fatigue.

Causes

Multifactorial and often unknown. There are risk factors that may predispose an individual to develop CRC (see Risk factors box).

Investigations

- Bowel Cancer Screening Programme: faecal occult blood test in men and women aged 60–69 years.
- Bloods: FBC for iron deficiency anaemia and carcinoembryonic antigen (CEA) tumour marker.
- Endoscopy: colonoscopy/sigmoidoscopy.
- Imaging: double contrast barium enema study 'apple core' sign; virtual colonoscopy.

Treatment

Depends on the extent of disease. This is assessed using Dukes' staging system or TNM system.

- Conservative: patient education and referral to Macmillan nurses.
- Medical: chemotherapy (oxaliplatin, folinic acid and 5-fluorouracil is the most common regimen); radiotherapy may also be used.
- Surgical: surgical resection is usually treatment of choice.

Complications

- Obstruction and metastasis.

Risk factors

- Smoking.
- Family history of CRC.
- *Streptococcus bovis* bacteraemia.
- Congenital polyposis syndromes:
  - Juvenile polyposis syndrome:
    - Autosomal dominant but it may occur spontaneously.
    - Not malignant.
  - Peutz–Jeghers syndrome:
    - Autosomal dominant.
    - Increases risk of CRC.
    - Melanosis is present on the oral mucosa.
- Genetic predisposition:
  - Familial adenomatous polyposis (FAP):
    - Autosomal dominant.
    - Mutation of *APC* gene on chromosome 5.
    - 100% lead to CRC.
  - Hereditary nonpolyposis colorectal cancer (HNPCC):
    - Autosomal dominant.
    - Mutation of DNA mismatch repair gene.
  - Amsterdam Criteria for HNPCC are a set list of criteria that help clinicians identify families at risk of HNPCC.
    It can be thought of as the 3-2-1 rule, as follows:
    - At least 3 relatives with histologically confirmed colorectal cancer, 1 of whom is a first degree relative of the other 2; familial adenomatous polyposis should be excluded.
    - At least 2 successive generations involved.
    - At least 1 of the cancers diagnosed before age 50.

- Increased age.
- Inflammatory bowel disease (IBD).

MAP 3.7 Colorectal Cancer (CRC)

TNM for CRC

Primary tumour staging

- Tx: primary tumour cannot be assessed.
- T0: no evidence of primary tumour.
- Tis: carcinoma in situ.
- T1: into (but not through) submucosa.
- T2: into (but not through) muscularis propria.
- T3: through muscularis propria into subserosa or into non-peritonealised pericolic/perirectal tissues.
- T4a: penetration of the visceral peritoneal layer.
- T4b: penetration or adhesion to adjacent organs.

Nodal status

- Nx: nodes cannot be assessed.
- N0: no evidence of nodal involvement.
- N1a: involvement of 1 regional node.
- N1b: involvement of 2–3 regional nodes.
- N1c: deposits involving serosa or non-peritonealised pericolic/perirectal tissues without regional nodal metastasis.
- N2a: involvement of 4–6 nodes.
- N2b: involvement of ≥7 nodes.

Metastases (M)

- Mx: presence of metastases cannot be assessed.
- M0: no evidence of metastases.
- M1a: distant metastases confined to one organ (e.g. liver, lung, ovary, non-regional node).
- M1b: distant metastases confined to more than one organ or to the peritoneum.

Dukes' staging system

Stage	Description	5-year survival rate (%)
A	Confined to muscularis mucosa	90
B	Through muscularis propria	65
C	Lymph node involvement	30
D	Distant metastases	<10

Map 3.7 Colorectal Cancer (CRC)

Map 3.8 Pancreatitis

MAP 3.8 **Pancreatitis**

ACUTE PANCREATITIS

What is acute pancreatitis?

This is inflammation of the pancreatic parenchyma, with biochemical associations of increased amylase and raised lipase enzymes on blood test.

Signs and symptoms

Remember these as **PAN**:

- Epigastric **P**ain that radiates to the back.
- **A**norexia.
- **N**ausea and vomiting.
- Grey Turner's sign: flank bruising.
- Cullen's sign: periumbilical bruising.

Causes

Remember these as **I GET SMASHED**:

- **I**diopathic.
- **G**allstones.
- **E**thanol.
- **T**rauma.
- **S**corpion sting (*Tityus trinitatis*).
- **M**umps.
- **A**utoimmune disease.
- **S**teroids.
- **H**yperlipidaemia/**H**ypercalcaemia.
- **E**ndoscopic retrograde cholangiopancreatography (ERCP).
- **D**rugs, e.g. azathioprine.

Investigations

- Bloods: FBC, U&Es, LFTs, Coag, calcium, LDH, amylase, lipase, CRP, glucose, ABG.
- Raised serum amylase and lipase.
- Detect cause, e.g. ultrasound scan to detect presence of gallstones.
  +/– MRCP (+/– ERCP to remove stones).
- CT scan to rule out complications (not within <72 h of acute presentation unless clinically indicated).

CHRONIC PANCREATITIS

What is chronic pancreatitis?

This is where the structural integrity of the pancreas is permanently altered as a direct result of chronic inflammation.

Signs and symptoms

Pain! The pain is:

- Epigastric in origin.
- Recurrent.
- Radiates to the back.
- Relieved by sitting forward.
- Worse when eating/drinking heavily.

Causes

Remember these as **CAMP**:

- **C**ystic fibrosis.
- **A**lcohol.
- **M**alnourishment.
- **P**ancreatic duct obstruction.

Investigations

- Decreased faecal elastase.
- CT scan: shows calcification (may also be seen on abdominal X-ray).
- Magnetic resonance cholangiopancreatography (MRCP).

Treatment

- This is usually symptomatic relief. Keep 'nil by mouth' (NBM), IV fluids and analgesia, e.g. tramadol
- Treat underlying causes, e.g. ERCP to remove gallstones.

Complications

Remember these as **HDAMN**:

- **H**aemorrhage.
- **D**isseminated intravascular coagulation (DIC).
- **A**cute respiratory distress syndrome (ARDS).
- **M**ultiorgan failure.
- **N**ecrosis.

Scoring systems

- Glasgow–Imrie criteria: remember as **PANCREAS**.
  - P – PaO₂ <7.9 kPa
  - A – Age >55 years
  - N – Neutrophils (WBC >15)
  - C – Calcium >2 mmol/L
  - R – Renal (serum urea >16 mmol/L)
  - E – Enzymes (LDH >600 IU/L)
  - A – Albumin <32 g/L
  - S – Sugar (glucose >10 mmol/L)
- Apache II score.

Treatment

- Conservative: alcohol cessation.
- Medical: analgesia, e.g. tramadol and pancreatic enzyme replacement therapy; start insulin therapy if diabetes has developed.

Complications

Remember these as **PODS**:

- **P**seudocysts.
- **O**bstruction (pancreatic).
- **D**iabetes mellitus.
- **S**teatorrhoea.

- Balthazar (CT scoring system) has 2 parts: 1. the grading of pancreatitis (A–E) and 2. the percentage of pancreatic necrosis. The maximum score that can be obtained is 10.
  - Grading of pancreatitis (Balthazar score).
    - A – normal pancreas: 0.
    - B – enlargement of pancreas: 1.
    - C – inflammatory changes in pancreas and peripancreatic fat: 2.
    - D – ill-defined single peripancreatic fluid collection: 3.
    - E – two or more poorly defined peripancreatic fluid collections: 4.
  - Pancreatic necrosis.
    - None: 0.
    - ≤30%: 2.
    - >30–50%: 4.
    - >50%: 6.

Table 3.1 Microbiology of the Gastrointestinal (GI) Tract

TABLE 3.1 **Microbiology of the Gastrointestinal (GI) Tract**

Organism	Illness caused	Other
Vibrio vulnificus	Food poisoning	Found in seafood; Gram-negative bacterium
Bacillus cereus	Food poisoning	Found in reheated rice; Gram-positive bacterium
Staphylococcus aureus	Food poisoning	Found in contaminated meat and mayonnaise; Gram-positive bacterium
Clostridium botulinum	Food poisoning	Found in poorly canned foods; Gram-positive bacterium
Escherichia coli O157:H7	Food poisoning and diarrhoea	Found in meat that is undercooked; enteropathogenic *E. coli* causes diarrhoea in children; also causes haemolytic uraemic syndrome (HUS); Gram-negative bacterium
Campylobacter jejuni	Bloody diarrhoea	Found in animal faeces and poultry; it is associated with Guillain–Barré syndrome, which is an ascending paralysis; Gram-negative bacterium
Salmonella	Bloody diarrhoea	Found in contaminated food; Gram-negative bacterium
Shigella	Bloody diarrhoea	Produces shiga toxin; Gram-negative bacterium
Yersinia enterocolitica	Bloody diarrhoea	Associated with outbreaks in nurseries; Gram-negative bacterium
Enterotoxic *Escherichia coli*	Travellers' diarrhoea	Travellers' diarrhoea is usually self-limiting; Gram-negative bacterium
Vibrio cholerae	Rice water diarrhoea	Produces cholera toxin; Gram-negative bacterium
Cryptosporidium	Cryptosporidiosis	Associated with AIDS patients; protozoon
Norwalk virus	Gastroenteritis	Most common viral cause of nausea and vomiting
Helicobacter pylori	Risk factors for peptic ulcers, gastritis and gastric adenocarcinoma	Produces urease; treat with 'triple therapy', i.e. a proton pump inhibitor (PPI) with either clarithromycin and amoxicillin or clarithromycin and metronidazole; Gram-negative bacterium
Toxoplasma gondii	Toxoplasmosis	Cysts are found in meat or cat faeces; causes brain abscesses in AIDS patients; protozoon
Taenia solium	Intestinal tapeworms	Found in undercooked pork; cestode

Figure 4.1 Nephron Physiology

FIGURE 4.1 Nephron Physiology

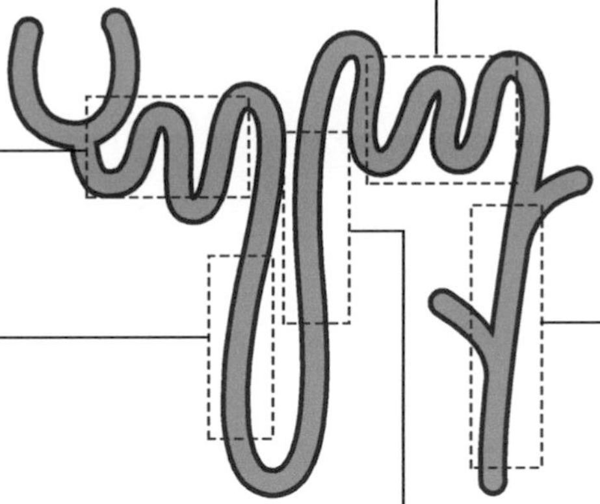

Proximal convoluted tubule
- Reabsorbs glucose, amino acids, water, bicarbonate ions, Na^+ and Cl^- ions
- Contains a brush border

Thin descending loop of Henle
- Reabsorbs water by medullary hypertonicity
- It is impermeable to Na^+ ions

Thick ascending loop of Henle
- Permeable to Na^+ ions
- Impermeable to water
- Contains the $Na^+/K^+/2Cl^-$ transporter

Distal convoluted tubule
- Actively reabsorbs Na^+ and Cl^- ions
- Simple cuboidal epithelium

Collecting tubule
- Aldosterone: increases the number of Na^+ ion channel in the collecting tubules
- Antidiuretic hormone (ADH): binds to V_2 receptors and consequently increases the number of aquaporins

FIGURE 4.2 **The Renin–Angiotensin–Aldosterone System (RAAS)**

Renin secretion is stimulated by:
- ↓ Blood pressure
- ↓ Na$^+$ ion and H$_2$O delivery to the macula densa
- ↑ Sympathetic activity

Angiotensinogen (LIVER)

Renin (KIDNEY)

Angiotensin I

Angiotensin converting enzyme (ACE) (LUNGS)

Angiotensin II

↑ Blood pressure by:
- Vasoconstriction of smooth muscle
- Stimulating aldosterone – ↑ Na$^+$ ion and H$_2$O retention
- Stimulating antidiuretic hormone (ADH) (posterior pituitary gland) – ↑ H$_2$O reabsorption
- ↑ Thirst by stimulating the hypothalamus

Figure 4.2 The Renin–Angiotensin–Aldosterone System (RAAS)

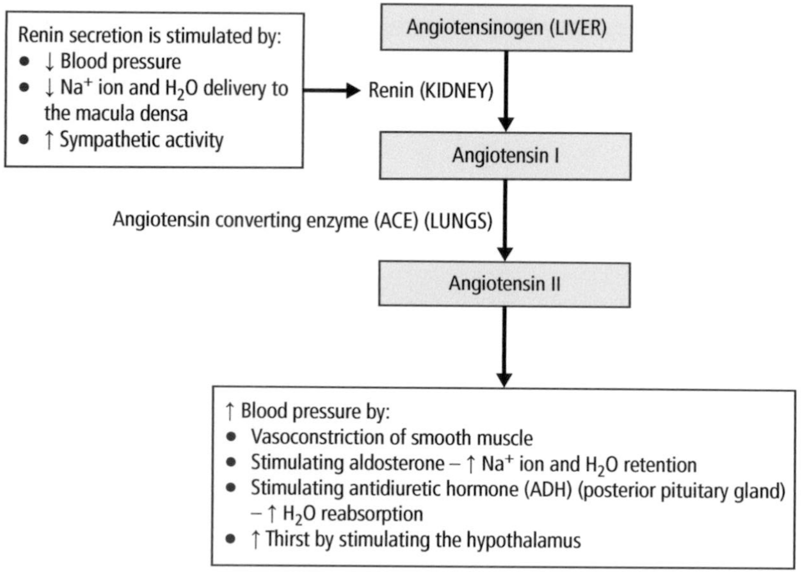

Table 4.1 Diuretics

TABLE 4.1 Diuretics

Class of diuretic	Example	Mechanism of action	Uses	Side effects	Contraindications	Drug interactions
Thiazide diuretic	Bendroflumethiazide	Blocks Na⁺/Cl⁻ ion symporter in the distal convoluted tubule	Hypertension Heart failure Ascites	Hyponatraemia Hypokalaemia Hypercalcaemia Hyperglycaemia Hyperlipidaemia Hyperuricaemia	Gout Liver failure Renal failure May worsen diabetes	Hypokalaemia may increase the risk of digoxin toxicity Decreased lithium excretion
Loop diuretic	Furosemide	Blocks Na⁺/K⁺/2Cl⁻ co-transporter in the ascending loop of Henle	Heart failure (symptomatic treatment of oedema) Severe hypercalcaemia	Hyponatraemia Hypokalaemia Hypocalcaemia Ototoxicity	Renal failure	Hypokalaemia may increase the risk of digoxin toxicity Decreased lithium excretion

K+-sparing diuretic	Spironolactone	Aldosterone receptor antagonist	Heart failure (in combination with furosemide) Oedema Ascites Refractory hypertension Conn's syndrome	Hyperkalaemia Gynaecomastia (alternatively, eplerenone can be given as a more selective aldosterone antagonist)	Addison's disease Hyperkalaemia	Decreased lithium excretion
Osmotic diuretic	Mannitol	Increases plasma osmolarity	Cerebral oedema Rhabdomyolysis Haemolysis	Fever Hyponatraemia	Heart failure	Increases levels of tobramycin

Table 4.1 Diuretics

Map 4.1 Renal Calculi

What are renal calculi?
These are stones that form within the renal tract.
Most stones are made from calcium (radiopaque), but others are made from struvite (staghorn calculus) and uric acid crystals (radiolucent).

Signs and symptoms
- Asymptomatic.
- Pain (suprapubic and loin pain that may radiate to the genital region).
- Dysuria.
- Urinary tract infection (UTI).
- Haematuria.

Investigations
- 24-h urine analysis: assess levels of calcium, uric acid, oxalate and citrate.
- CT kidney, ureter, bladder (KUB): for radiopaque stones.
- Ultrasound and IVU can also be utilised.
- Chemical analysis of stone composition.

MAP 4.1 **Renal Calculi**

Causes
- Idiopathic.
- Hypercalcaemia.
- Hyperuricaemia.
- Hyperoxaluria.
- Recurrent UTI.
- Drugs, e.g. loop diuretics.
- Hereditary conditions increase risk, e.g. polycystic kidney disease.

Complications
- Recurrent UTI.
- Recurrent calculi.
- Obstruction.
- Trauma to ureter/ureteric stricture.

Treatment

- Conservative: prevent cause, e.g. low calcium diet. Education about risk factors.
- Medical: in adults, organise follow-up in urology stone clinic as per trust policy but generally:

Ureteric stone <5 mm	Consider watchful waiting for asymptomatic renal stones in adults, children and young people
Ureteric stone <10 mm	Consider SWL Consider URS if there are contraindications for SWL, or the stone is not targetable with SWL, or a previous course of SWL has failed
Ureteric stone 10–20 mm	Offer URS Consider SWL if local facilities allow up to 2 SWL sessions within 4 weeks of the decision to treat Consider PCNL for impacted proximal stones when URS has failed
Renal stone <10 mm	Offer SWL Consider URS if there are contraindications for SWL, or a previous course of SWL has failed, or because of anatomical reasons, SWL is not indicated Consider PCNL if SWL and URS have failed to treat the current stone or are not an option
Renal stone 10–20 mm	Consider URS or SWL Consider PCNL if URS or SWL have failed
Renal stone >20 mm, incl. staghorn stones	Offer PCNL Consider URS if PCNL is not an option

- Radiology:
  - Nephrostomy insertion.
  - Antegrade ureteric stent insertion.
- Surgical:
  - Antegrade or retrograde removal of large stones or staghorn calculus.
  - Extracorporeal shock wave lithotripsy (ESWL) for the treatment of larger stones (>0.5 cm).

Map 4.1 Renal Calculi

Map 4.2 Urinary Tract Infection (UTI)

What is a UTI?

This is an infection of the urinary tract with typical signs and symptoms. It may be classified as either a lower or upper (acute pyelonephritis) UTI.

Signs and symptoms of lower UTI

- Dysuria.
- Frequency.
- Urgency.
- Suprapubic pain.
- Lower back pain.

Signs and symptoms of upper UTI

- Fever/chills.
- Flank pain.
- Haematuria.

Risk factors

- Female gender.
- Sexual intercourse.
- Catheterisation.
- Pregnancy.
- Menopause.
- Diabetes.
- Genitourinary malformation.
- Immunosuppression.
- Urinary tract obstruction, e.g. stones.

Pathophysiology

The urinary system has many defences to prevent UTI such as:

- Micturition.
- Urine: osmolarity, pH and organic acids are antibacterial.
- Secreted factors:
  - Tamm–Horsfall protein: binds bacteria non-specifically; produced by cells of the thick ascending loop of Henle; mutations in the gene that codes for this protein are associated with progressive renal failure and medullary cysts.
  - IgA: against specific bacteria.
  - Lactoferrin: hoovers up free iron.
- Mucosal defences: mucopolysaccharides coat the mucosal surfaces of the bladder.
- If these defence mechanisms are overcome by bacterial virulence factors then the patient is prone to developing a UTI. Some virulence factors worth noting are:
- For uropathogenic E. coli (UPEC):
  - Type 1 fimbriae: binds to mannose residues; associated with cystitis.
  - Type P fimbriae: binds to glycolipid residues; associated with pyelonephritis.
  - Bacterial capsule: aka antigen K, resists phagocytosis; associated with pyelonephritis.
- For Proteus mirabilis:
  - Produces urease.
  - Increases pH of urine.
  - Proteus mirabilis is associated with staghorn calculi.

MAP 4.2 **Urinary Tract Infection (UTI)**

Causative organisms

- *Escherichia coli*: leading cause of UTI in the community and also nosocomial infection. Metallic sheen on eosin methylene blue (EMB).
- *Staphylococcus saprophyticus*: 2nd leading cause in sexually active females.
- *Klebsiella pneumoniae*: 3rd leading cause. Viscous colonies.
- *Proteus mirabilis*: produces urease. Gram-negative bacterium.
- *Pseudomonas aeruginosa*: bile green pigment and fruity odour. Usually nosocomial and drug resistant.
- Adenovirus: haemorrhagic cystitis.
- BK and JC viruses: associated with graft failure after transplantation.
- *Schistosoma haematobium*: parasitic infection.

Investigations

- Urine dipstick: positive for leucocytes and nitrites.
- Urine culture: for diagnosis for causative organism ($>10^5$ organisms per mL of midstream urine).
- Radiology: consider ultrasound scan or cystoscopy if UTI occurs in children, in men or if UTI is recurrent.

Treatment

- Conservative: education about the condition and avoidance of predisposing risk factors.
- Medical: treat with antibiotics as per local guidelines. This typically will be a course of trimethoprim or nitrofurantoin of variable length depending on whether the patient is male or female.
- If recurrent, i.e. >4 UTIs per year, seek to exclude anatomical variant or abnormality of the renal tract.

Complications

- Pyelonephritis.
- Renal failure.
- Sepsis.

Map 4.2 Urinary Tract Infection (UTI)

Map 4.3 Renal Cancers

MAP 4.3 **Renal Cancers**

RENAL CELL CARCINOMA (RCC)
What is RCC?
This is an adenocarcinoma originating from the cells that line the proximal convoluted tubule.

Risk factors
● Male.
● Age 50–70 years.
● Smoking.
● Obesity.
● Mutation of the Von Hippel–Lindau tumour suppressor gene on chromosome 3.

Signs and symptoms
● Unintentional weight loss.
● Loin pain.
● Haematuria.
● Palpable mass.
● Fever.
● Hypertension.

TRANSITIONAL CELL CARCINOMA (TCC)
What is TCC?
This is a cancer that arises from transitional urothelium. It is more common in men.

Risk factors
Remember these as **CAPS**:
● **C**yclophosphamide.
● **A**niline dyes.
● **P**henacetin.
● **S**moking.

Signs and symptoms
Depends on the location of the cancer but is usually associated with painless haematuria and lower urinary tract symptoms, e.g. frequency and urgency.

Paraneoplastic syndromes involved

- Secretion of adrenocorticotrophic hormone (ACTH): may produce symptoms of hypercalcaemia.
- Secretion of erythropoietin (EPO): may produce symptoms of polycythaemia.

Investigations

- Radiology (ultrasound scan, CT scan, MRI scan).

Treatment

- Conservative: patient education. Supportive, counselling and monitoring of psychological wellbeing (depression). Refer patients to Macmillan nurses.
- Medical: interferon-alpha, sunitinib, sorafenib, bevacizumab.
- Surgical: partial or total nephrectomy is the treatment of choice; radiofrequency ablation may be considered.

Complications

- Metastasis: to brain, bone, lung, liver, adrenal glands and lymph nodes.
- Hypercalcaemia.
- Hypertension.
- Polycythaemia.

Investigations

- Cystoscopy and ureteroscopy with biopsy.
- Retrograde pyelography.
- CT scan.
- MRI scan.

Treatment

- Conservative: supportive counselling and monitoring of psychological wellbeing (depression). Refer patients to Macmillan nurses.
- Medical: mitomycin, GC regimen (gemcitabine and cisplatin) or MVAC regimen (methotrexate, vinblastine, doxorubicin and cisplatin).
- Surgical: nephroureterectomy, cystectomy; radiofrequency ablation may be considered.

Complications

- Metastasis, usually to bone.

Map 4.3 Renal Cancers

Map 4.4 Kidney Injury

MAP 4.4 Kidney Injury

ACUTE KIDNEY INJURY (AKI)

What is AKI?

This is when the kidney fails over a short time period (days to weeks) and is characterised by a rapid fall in glomerular filtration rate (GFR) and an increase in creatinine and urea levels. It may be reversible. AKI may be subdivided into prerenal, intrinsic renal and postrenal failure and these have many different causes.

According to NICE, AKI can be detected using any of the following criteria:

- A rise in serum creatinine of ≥26 μmol/L within 48 hours.
- A ≥50% rise in serum creatinine known or presumed to have occurred within the past 7 days.
- A fall in urine output to <0.5 mL/kg/h for more than 6 hours.

Causes

Prerenal	Intrinsic	Postrenal
Hypovolaemia	Glomerular disease	Obstruction of the ureter
• Haemorrhage	• Glomerulonephritis	• Stones
• Burns	• Vasculitis	• Tumour
• Diuretic use	• Immune complex disease, e.g. systemic lupus erythematosus (SLE)	
Shock	Vascular lesions	Obstruction of the bladder neck
• Sepsis	• Bilateral renal artery stenosis	• Stones
• Cardiogenic	• Microangiopathy	• Tumour
	• Malignant hypertension	• Benign prostatic hypertrophy
		• Prostate cancer

CHRONIC KIDNEY INJURY (CKI)

What is CKI?

This is well-established renal impairment and is irreversible. Renal function progressively worsens with time. Without treatment the patient will eventually develop end-stage kidney disease (ESKD).

Causes

- Any renal disease may lead to CKI.
- Glomerulonephritis.
- Hypertension.
- Diabetes mellitus.
- Malignancy.
- Anatomical abnormality of the renal tract.
- Hereditary disease, e.g. polycystic kidney disease.

Signs and symptoms

Oliguria/anuria/polyuria, nausea and vomiting, confusion, hypertension, oedema (peripheral and pulmonary), fatigue, metallic taste in mouth, unintentional weight loss, itchy skin, skin pigmentation, Kussmaul breathing (metabolic acidosis), anaemia.

Hypoperfusion	Tubulointerstitial disease	Obstruction of the urethra
• Hepatorenal syndrome • NSAID use • Angiotensin converting enzyme (ACE) inhibitor use	• Acute tubular necrosis • Acute tubulointerstitial nephritis • Multiple myeloma • Nephrotoxic drugs	• Tumour • Stricture
Oedematous conditions • Heart failure • Nephrotic syndrome		

Signs and symptoms

Oliguria/anuria, nausea and vomiting, confusion, hypertension, abdominal/flank pain, signs of fluid overload, e.g. ↑ jugular venous pressure (JVP).

Investigations

- GFR.
- Bloods: FBC and platelets, U&Es, creatinine, calcium and phosphate levels, ESR, CRP, immunology, virology.
- Urinalysis: blood, protein, glucose, leucocytes and nitrites, Bence Jones protein.
- Imaging: ultrasound scan.

Treatment

- Maintain renal blood flow and fluid balance.
- Monitor electrolytes.
- Treat underlying cause; classify AKI with **RIFLE** criteria (**R**isk, **I**njury, **F**ailure, **L**oss, **E**nd-stage renal disease).
- Stop all nephrotoxic drugs.

Complications

- Metabolic acidosis.
- Hyperkalaemia.
- Hyperphosphataemia.
- Pulmonary oedema.

Investigations

- GFR.
- Bloods: FBC, U&Es, creatinine, calcium and phosphate levels, ESR, CRP, immunology, virology.
- Urinalysis: blood, protein, glucose, leucocytes and nitrites; Bence Jones proteinuria (multiple myeloma).
- Imaging: ultrasound scan.
- Renal biopsy.

Treatment

- Conservative: smoking cessation, low salt diet, maintain psychological wellbeing.
- Medical:
  - Treat underlying cause and complications.
    - Control blood pressure.
    - Treat anaemia.
    - Treat acidosis (with sodium bicarbonate).
    - Treat hyperphosphataemia (with phosphate binders).
- Surgical: dialysis (haemodialysis or peritoneal dialysis), renal transplantation.

Complications

- Anaemia.
- Hypertension.
- Renal bone disease.
- Metabolic acidosis.
- Stroke.
- Peripheral nerve damage.
- Carpal tunnel syndrome.
- Oedematous states.
- Depression.

Map 4.4 Kidney Injury

Map 4.5 Nephritic vs. Nephrotic Syndrome

NEPHRITIC SYNDROME

What is nephritic syndrome?

This is a group of signs of varying diseases.

Signs

Remember these as **PHARAOH**:

- **P**roteinuria.
- **H**aematuria.
- **A**zotaemia.
- **R**ed blood cell casts.
- **A**ntistreptolysin O titres.
- **O**liguria.
- **H**ypertension.

Causes

These may be split broadly into 2 categories: focal proliferative and diffuse proliferative causes.

Focal proliferative	Diffuse proliferative
IgA nephropathy	Rapidly progressive glomerulonephritis, e.g. Goodpasture's syndrome
Systemic lupus erythematosus (SLE)	SLE
Henoch–Schönlein purpura	Membranoproliferative glomerulonephritis
Alport's syndrome	Cryoglobulinaemia

MAP 4.5 Nephritic vs. Nephrotic Syndrome

NEPHROTIC SYNDROME

What is nephrotic syndrome?

This is a group of signs of varying diseases.

Signs

Remember these as **PHHO**:

- **P**roteinuria >3 g daily.
- **H**ypoalbuminaemia <30 g/L.
- **H**yperlipidaemia, occurs because:
  - Hypoproteinaemia stimulates the production of more proteins from the liver, which results in the synthesis of more lipoproteins.
  - Decreased levels of lipoprotein lipase means that lipid catabolism decreases.
- **O**edema.

Causes

- Minimal change disease.
- Focal segmental glomerulosclerosis.
- Membranous glomerulonephritis.
- Diabetic nephropathy.
- Amyloidosis.

Investigations

- Bloods: FBC, WCC and platelets, U&Es, LFTs, creatinine, urea, CRP, ESR, glucose, lipid profile.
- Urinalysis: blood, protein, glucose, leucocytes, nitrites and Bence Jones protein.
- Nephritic screen: serum complement (C3 and C4), antinuclear antibody (ANA), double stranded DNA (dsDNA), antineutrophil cytoplasmic antibody (ANCA), antiglomerular basement membrane (anti-GBM), HIV serology, HBV and HCV serology, blood cultures, Venereal Disease Research Laboratory Test (VDRL) for syphilis.
- Renal biopsy.
- Radiology: ultrasound scan.

Treatment

- Conservative: lifestyle advice, low salt diet.
- Medical: treatment depends on cause:
  o Treat hypertension.
  o Treat proteinuria.
  o Treat hypercholesterolaemia.
  o Give prophylactic anticoagulation therapy.
  o Immunotherapy regimen, e.g. prednisolone, cyclophosphamide and azathioprine.
  o Dialysis if severe.

Complications

- Nephrotic syndrome.
- Chronic glomerulonephritis.
- Heart failure.

- Mesangial proliferative glomerulonephritis.
- SLE.

Investigations

- Bloods: FBC, WCC and platelets, U&Es, LFTs, creatinine, urea, CRP, ESR, glucose, lipid profile.
- Urinalysis: blood, protein, glucose, leucocytes, nitrites and Bence Jones protein.
- Nephritic screen: serum complement (C3 and C4), ANA, dsDNA, ANCA, anti-GBM, HIV serology, HBV and HCV serology, blood cultures, VDRL for syphilis.
- Renal biopsy.
- Radiology: ultrasound scan.

Treatment

- Conservative: lifestyle advice, low salt diet.
- Medical: treatment depends on cause:
  o Treat hypertension.
  o Treat proteinuria.
  o Treat hypercholesterolaemia.
  o Give prophylactic anticoagulation therapy.
  o Immunotherapy regimen, e.g. prednisolone, cyclophosphamide and azathioprine.
  o Dialysis if severe.

Complications

- Hypertension.
- Acute kidney injury.
- Chronic kidney injury.
- Infection.

Map 4.5 Nephritic vs. Nephrotic Syndrome

Map 4.6 Cystic Disease

ADPKD

What is ADPKD?

This is a dominantly inherited polycystic disease found in adults.

Causes

Mutations in the genes encoding a membrane protein called polycystin result in this condition. Two genes code for this protein:

- *PKD1* on chromosome 16 (encodes polycystin 1).
- *PKD2* on chromosome 4 (encodes polycystin 2).

Signs and symptoms

- Pain (due to renal cyst haemorrhage).
- Hypertension.
- Haematuria.
- Palpable bilateral flank masses.
- Hepatomegaly.

Investigations

- Bloods: FBC, U&Es, calcium and phosphate, PTH.
- Urinalysis and culture.
- Imaging: ultrasound scan is diagnostic.
- Genetic screening and monitoring of blood pressure.

Remember cystic disease as CAAR:

- **C**ystic renal dysplasia.
- **A**utosomal dominant polycystic kidney disease (ADPKD).
- **A**utosomal recessive polycystic kidney disease (ARPKD).
- **C**ystic diseases of the **R**enal medulla.

MAP 4.6
Cystic Disease

ARPKD

What is ARPKD?

This is a recessively inherited polycystic disease found in children presenting with varying levels of kidney and liver disease.

Causes

- *PKHD1* on chromosome 6.

Signs and symptoms

- Hypertension.
- Those of chronic kidney injury.
- Chronic respiratory infections.
- Those of portal hypertension: ascites, caput medusae and oesophageal varices.
- Failure to thrive.
- Recurrent UTI.
- Polyuria.

Investigations

- Antenatal screening is diagnostic.
- Bloods: FBC, U&Es, LFTs.
- Urinalysis and culture.
- Imaging: ultrasound scan (shows enlarged kidney with or without oligohydramnios), CT scan, MRI scan.

Treatment

- Conservative: parental and patient support.
- Medical:
  - Ventilation and long-term oxygen therapy.
  - Treat hypertension (angiotensin converting enzyme [ACE] inhibitors).
  - Antibiotics for UTI.
  - Diuretics for fluid overload.
- Surgical:
  - Nephrectomy.
  - Combined renal and liver transplantation.

Complications

- Hepatic cysts.
- Congenital hepatic fibrosis.
- Proliferative bile ducts.

Cystic diseases of the renal medulla

Remember **NAMS**:

- **N**ephronophthisis medullary cystic disease.
- **A**cquired cystic disease: usually from dialysis.
- **M**edullary sponge kidney.
- **S**imple cysts.

Treatment

- Conservative: patient support.
- Medical:
  - Treat hypertension.
  - Antibiotic therapy for urinary tract infection (UTI).
- Surgical: cyst decompression.

Complications

- Development of chronic kidney injury.
- Remember **LAMB**:
  - **L**iver cysts.
  - **A**neurysms.
  - **M**itral valve prolapse.
  - **B**erry aneurysm rupture leading to subarachnoid haemorrhage.

Map 4.6 Cystic Disease

Map 4.7 Congenital Kidney Abnormalities

HORSESHOE KIDNEY
What is a horseshoe kidney?
This occurs during development when the lower poles of both kidneys fuse, resulting in the formation of one horseshoe-shaped kidney. This cannot ascend to the normal anatomical position due to the central fused portion catching the inferior mesenteric artery.

Signs and symptoms
- Asymptomatic.
- Recurrent urinary tract infection (UTI).
- Renal calculi.
- Obstructive uropathy.

Causes
- Congenital abnormality.

Investigations
- Ultrasound scan is diagnostic.

Treatment
- Treatment of complications.

Complications
- Susceptible to trauma.
- Renal calculi formation.
- Increased risk of transitional cell carcinoma of the renal pelvis.

ECTOPIC KIDNEY
What is an ectopic kidney?
This is a congenital abnormality in which the kidney lies above the pelvic brim or within the pelvis.

Signs and symptoms
- Usually asymptomatic.

Causes
- Genetic abnormalities.
- Poor development of the metanephrogenic diverticulum.
- Teratogen exposure.

Investigations
- Ultrasound scan is diagnostic.

Treatment
- None; treat complications should they develop.

Complications
- UTI.
- Renal calculi.

Remember these as HERD:
- **H**orseshoe kidney.
- **E**ctopic kidney.
- **R**enal agenesis.
- **D**uplex ureters.

MAP 4.7 Congenital Kidney Abnormalities

DUPLEX URETERS

What are duplex ureters?

This occurs when the ureteric bud splits during embryonic development and results in the development of 2 ureters, which drain 1 kidney.

Signs and symptoms

- Asymptomatic.
- Recurrent UTI.

Causes

- Splitting of the ureteric bud.

Investigations

- Ultrasound scan and excretory urography is diagnostic.

Treatment

- Treatment of complications.

Complications

- Vesicoureteral reflux.
- Ureterocele.
- UTI.

RENAL AGENESIS

What is renal agenesis?

Bilateral or unilateral absence of the kidney.

Signs and symptoms

Bilateral absence (Potter's syndrome)	Unilateral absence
Low-set ears	Hypertension
Limb defects	Increased risk of respiratory infections
Receding chin	Proteinuria
Flat, broad nose	Haematuria

Causes

- Failure of ureteric bud development.

Investigations

- Antenatal screening.

Treatment

This depends on whether there is bilateral or unilateral absence of the kidney.

Bilateral absence (Potter's syndrome)	Unilateral absence
Neonates usually die a few days after birth. If the baby survives they require chronic peritoneal dialysis	Treatment of hypertension

Complications

- Susceptible to trauma (unilateral).
- Death.

Map 4.7 Congenital Kidney Abnormalities

Map 5.1 Hyperthyroidism

What is hyperthyroidism?

This occurs when there is too much circulating thyroid hormone in the body.
There are many different causes of hyperthyroidism.

Causes

Cause	Comment
Graves' disease	• This is the most common cause of hyperthyroidism • It is an autoimmune condition • May be distinguished from other causes of hyperthyroidism by ocular changes, e.g. exophthalmos, and other signs, e.g. pretibial myxoedema • It is associated with other autoimmune conditions such as pernicious anaemia • Graves' disease is caused by thyroid-stimulating immunoglobulin (TSI), also known as thyroid-stimulating antibody (TSAb). Thyroid-stimulating immunoglobulin binds with thyroid-stimulating hormone (TSH) receptor on the thyroid cell membrane and stimulates the action of the thyroid-stimulating hormone
Toxic multinodular goitre and toxic solitary nodule goitre	• This is the second most common cause of hyperthyroidism • Risk increases with age • More common in females • A single nodule is suggestive of thyroid neoplasia
De Quervain's thyroiditis	• This is transient hyperthyroidism that develops after a viral infection • Goitre is often painful • A period of hypothyroidism may follow

Signs and symptoms

- Weight loss.
- Warm skin/heat intolerance.
- Diarrhoea.
- Exophthalmos (Graves' disease).
- Lid lag.
- Palpitations.
- Anxiety.
- Tremor.
- Goitre +/– bruit.
- Brisk reflexes.

MAP 5.1
Hyperthyroidism

Investigations

- TFTs ($\downarrow$ TSH, $\uparrow T_3$, and $\uparrow T_4$).
- Ultrasound scan of nodules.
- Fine needle aspiration of solitary nodules to exclude malignancy.
- Isotope scan to assess hot and cold thyroid nodules.

Treatment

- Conservative: patient education, smoking cessation.
- Medical:

Symptomatic control	Palpitations and tremor: beta-blockers Eye symptoms: eye drops for lubrication
Antithyroid medication	Carbimazole Propylthiouracil Side effects: agranulocytosis (monitor patient's bloods carefully)
Radioactive iodine ablation	Definitive treatment; patients must be euthyroid before commencing treatment

- Surgical: subtotal thyroidectomy, patients must be euthyroid before the procedure. Give the patient potassium iodide before surgery since it decreases thyroid gland vascularity.

Complications

- Atrial fibrillation.
- High output heart failure.
- Cardiomyopathy.
- Osteoporosis.

Map 5.1 Hyperthyroidism

What is hypothyroidism?

This occurs when there is too little circulating thyroid hormone in the body. There are many different causes of hypothyroidism.

Causes	
Type of hypothyroidism	**Cause**
Primary hypothyroidism	• Iodine deficiency • Hashimoto's autoimmune thyroiditis • Post-thyroidectomy/radioactive iodine therapy • Drug induced, e.g. lithium, overtreatment of hyperthyroidism
Secondary hypothyroidism	• Dysfunction of the hypothalamic–pituitary axis • Pituitary adenoma • Sheehan's syndrome (ischaemic necrosis of the pituitary gland after childbirth) • Infiltrative disease, e.g. tuberculosis and haemochromatosis

MAP 5.2 **Hypothyroidism**

Complications
- Hypercholesterolaemia.
- Complications in pregnancy, e.g. pre-eclampsia.
- Hyperthyroidism from overtreatment of hypothyroidism.
- Myxoedema coma.

Treatment
- Conservative: patient education.
- Medical: lifelong replacement of thyroid hormone with levothyroxine.

Investigations
- TFTs ($\uparrow$ TSH, $\downarrow$ T$_3$ and $\downarrow$ T$_4$).
- Thyroid antibodies.
- FBC (anaemia).
- U&Es.
- LFTs.
- Creatinine.
- Cholesterol.
- Guthrie test for congenital screening.

Signs and symptoms
- Weight gain.
- Cold skin/cold intolerance.
- Constipation.
- Dry skin.
- Thinning of hair.
- Bradycardia.
- Depression.
- Delayed reflexes.

Map 5.3 Thyroid Carcinoma

What is thyroid carcinoma?

This is cancer that originates from follicular or parafollicular cells.

Causes

Malignant neoplasm. Increased risk with childhood neck irradiation.

Thyroid carcinomas may be classified histopathologically.

Histological appearance	Percentage of thyroid cancer	Comment
Papillary	70	• Affects younger patients • Spreads to cervical lymph nodes	• Good prognosis
Follicular	20	• More common in low iodine areas • Spreads to bone and lungs	• Good prognosis • Haematogenous spread
Medullary	5	• Arises from parafollicular cells • Calcitonin is a biochemical marker	• Associated with MEN syndrome • Spreads to lymph nodes
Anaplastic	<5	• Affects older patients • Aggressive	• Spreads to lymph nodes • Poor prognosis
Other	–	• Lymphoma of the thyroid • Sarcoma of the thyroid	• Hürthle cell carcinoma (a variant of follicular carcinoma)

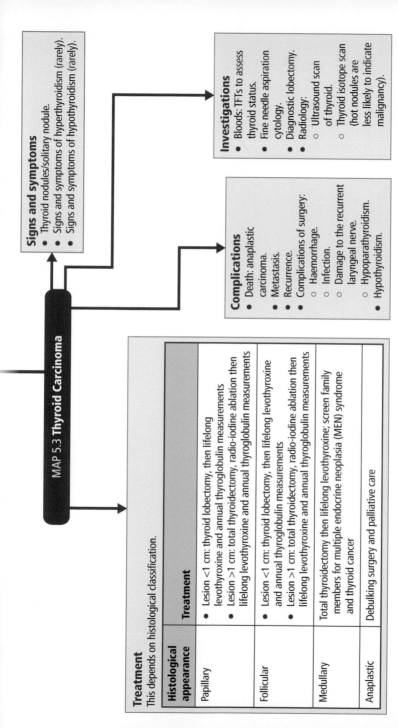

Signs and symptoms

- Thyroid nodules/solitary nodule.
- Signs and symptoms of hyperthyroidism (rarely).
- Signs and symptoms of hypothyroidism (rarely).

Investigations

- Bloods: TFTs to assess thyroid status.
- Fine needle aspiration cytology.
- Diagnostic lobectomy.
- Radiology:
  - Ultrasound scan of thyroid.
  - Thyroid isotope scan (hot nodules are less likely to indicate malignancy).

Complications

- Death: anaplastic carcinoma.
- Metastasis.
- Recurrence.
- Complications of surgery:
  - Haemorrhage.
  - Infection.
  - Damage to the recurrent laryngeal nerve.
  - Hypoparathyroidism.
- Hypothyroidism.

MAP 5.3 Thyroid Carcinoma

Treatment

This depends on histological classification.

Histological appearance	Treatment
Papillary	• Lesion <1 cm: thyroid lobectomy, then lifelong levothyroxine and annual thyroglobulin measurements • Lesion >1 cm: total thyroidectomy, radio-iodine ablation then lifelong levothyroxine and annual thyroglobulin measurements
Follicular	• Lesion <1 cm: thyroid lobectomy, then lifelong levothyroxine and annual thyroglobulin measurements • Lesion >1 cm: total thyroidectomy, radio-iodine ablation then lifelong levothyroxine and annual thyroglobulin measurements
Medullary	Total thyroidectomy then lifelong levothyroxine; screen family members for multiple endocrine neoplasia (MEN) syndrome and thyroid cancer
Anaplastic	Debulking surgery and palliative care

Map 5.3 Thyroid Carcinoma

Map 5.4 Diabetes Mellitus (DM)

What is DM?

This is a metabolic condition in which the patient has hyperglycaemia due to insulin insensitivity or decreased insulin secretion.

- Type 1 DM: this is an autoimmune condition, which results in the destruction of the pancreatic beta cells resulting in no insulin production. This condition has a juvenile onset and is associated with HLA-DR3 and HLA-DR4. Patients are at risk of ketoacidosis.
- Type 2 DM: this occurs when patients gradually become insulin resistant or when the pancreatic beta cells fail to secrete enough insulin or both. It usually has a later life onset; however, the incidence is increasing in young populations due to environmental factors such as increasing obesity and sedentary lifestyle. Patients are at risk of developing a hyperosmolar state.
- Other cause of DM include: chronic pancreatitis, gestational DM and cystic fibrosis.

Treatment

Treatment	Type 1 DM	Type 2 DM
Conservative	Dietary advice BMI measurement Smoking cessation Decrease alcohol intake Regular blood glucose and HbA1c monitoring Encourage exercise	Dietary advice: high in complex carbohydrates, low in fat BMI measurement Smoking cessation Decrease alcohol intake Regular blood glucose and HbA1c monitoring Encourage exercise
Medical	See pages 88–90 for antidiabetic agents	See pages 88–90 for antidiabetic agents

MAP 5.4 **Diabetes Mellitus (DM)**

Investigations

Diagnostic investigations include:
- Fasting plasma glucose: >7 mmol/L (126 mg/dL).
- Random plasma glucose (plus DM symptoms): >11.1 mmol/L (200 mg/dL).
- HbA1c: >6.5% (48 mmol/mol).

Other tests include:
- Impaired glucose tolerance test (for borderline cases):
  - Fasting plasma glucose: <7 mmol/L (126 mg/dL) and at 2 h, after a 75 g oral glucose load, a level of 7.8–11 mmol/L (140–200 mg/dL).
  - Plasma glucose at 2 h: >11.1 mmol/L (>200 mg/dL).
- Impaired fasting glucose: plasma glucose: 5.6–6.9 mmol/L (110–126 mg/dL).

Signs and symptoms

- General: polyuria, polyphagia, polydipsia, blurred vision, glycosuria, signs of macrovascular and microvascular disease.
- More common in type 1 DM: acetone breath, weight loss, Kussmaul breathing, nausea and vomiting.

Complications

- Macrovascular: hypertension, increased risk of stroke, myocardial infarction, diabetic foot.
- Microvascular: nephropathy, peripheral neuropathy (glove-and-stocking distribution), retinopathy, erectile dysfunction.
- Psychological: depression.

Table 5.1 Antidiabetic Agents

TABLE 5.1 **Antidiabetic Agents**

For a full description of diabetes mellitus (DM) management and which drugs to use first line, please follow the website link provided for NICE guidelines in Appendix Two

Class of antidiabetic agent	Example	Mechanism of action	Uses	Side effects	Contraindications	Drug interactions
Biguanides	Metformin	↑ Peripheral insulin sensitivity ↑ Glucose uptake into and use by skeletal muscle ↓ Hepatic gluconeogenesis ↓ Intestinal glucose absorption	Type 2 DM (first choice in overweight patients) Polycystic ovarian syndrome	Gastrointestinal tract (GIT) disturbance, e.g. diarrhoea Nausea Vomiting Lactic acidosis	Renal failure Cardiac failure Respiratory failure Hepatic failure (The above increase the risk of developing lactic acidosis)	Contrast agents Angiotensin converting enzyme (ACE) inhibitors Alcohol Nonsteroidal anti-inflammatory drugs (NSAIDs) Steroids
Sulphonylureas	Glipizide	Block potassium channels on the pancreatic beta cells, thus stimulating insulin release	Type 2 DM	GIT disturbance Hypoglycaemia Weight gain	Renal failure Hepatic failure Porphyria Pregnancy Breastfeeding	ACE inhibitors Alcohol NSAIDs Steroids
Meglitinides (glinides)	Repaglinide	Block potassium channels on the pancreatic beta cells, thus stimulating insulin release	Type 2 DM	Weight gain Hypoglycaemia	Hepatic failure Pregnancy Breastfeeding	Ciclosporin Trimethoprim Clarithromycin

Thiazolidinediones (glitazones)	Pioglitazone	Activates nuclear peroxisome proliferator activated receptor (PPAR)	Type 2 DM	Weight gain Hypoglycaemia Hepatotoxicity Fracture risk	Type 1 DM Hepatic disease Heart failure Bladder cancer	Rifampicin Paclitaxel
Incretins	Exenatide	Analogue of glucagon-like peptide (GLP)-1	Type 2 DM	GIT disturbance, e.g. diarrhoea Acute pancreatitis	Thyroid cancer Multiple endocrine neoplasia (MEN) 2 syndrome	Bexarotene
	Saxagliptin	Inhibits dipeptidyl peptidase (DPP)-4	Type 2 DM	GIT disturbance, e.g. diarrhoea Infection of the respiratory and urinary tracts Hepatotoxicity Peripheral oedema	History of serious hypersensitivity reaction	Thiazolidinedione
Sodium–glucose co-transporter-2 (SGLT2) inhibitors	Canagliflozin, dapagliflozin, empagliflozin	Inhibits SGLT2	Type 2 DM	Genital mycotic infections Urinary tract infections and increased urination Dizziness Dyslipidaemia Hypoglycaemia. Very rarely, angioedema and Fournier's gangrene	Type 1 DM (high risk of diabetic ketoacidosis)	Dapagliflozin

Continued overleaf

Table 5.1 Antidiabetic Agents

Table 5.1 Antidiabetic Agents

TABLE 5.1 **Antidiabetic Agents** (*Continued*)

Class of antidiabetic agent	Example	Mechanism of action	Uses	Side effects	Contraindications	Drug interactions
Alpha-glucosidase inhibitors	Acarbose	Inhibits alpha-glucosidase	Type 2 DM	GIT disturbance, e.g. diarrhoea	Inflammatory bowel disease (IBD) Intestinal obstruction Hepatic cirrhosis	Orlistat Pancreatin
Amylin analogues	Pramlintide	Analogue of amylin	Type 1 DM Type 2 DM	Severe hypoglycaemia	Gastroparesis Hypersensitivity to pramlintide	Acarbose
Insulin therapy	Rapid acting, e.g. insulin lispro Short acting, e.g. soluble insulin Intermediate acting, e.g. isophane insulin Long acting, e.g. insulin glargine Biphasic, e.g. biphasic isophane insulin	Replaces insulin *Mechanism of action of insulin:* Insulin binds to tyrosine kinase receptors where it initiates 2 pathways by phosphorylation: 1 The MAP kinase signalling pathway: this is responsible for cell growth and proliferation. 2 The PI-3K signalling pathway: this is responsible for the transport of GLUT-4 receptors to the cell surface membrane; GLUT-4 transports glucose into the cell; this pathway is also responsible for protein, lipid and glycogen synthesis	Type 1 DM Type 2 DM	Weight gain Hypoglycaemia Localised lipoatrophy Hypokalaemia	Hypersensitivity to any of the therapy ingredients Hypoglycaemia	Repaglinide increases risk of myocardial infarction (MI) and hypoglycaemia Monoamine oxidase inhibitors may increase insulin secretion Corticosteroids decrease the effect of insulin Levothyroxine decreases the effect of insulin Thiazide diuretics decrease the effects of insulin

What is DI?

A disorder caused by low levels of or insensitivity to antidiuretic hormone (ADH) leading to polyuria. This can be cranial or nephrogenic in origin.

Causes

- Cranial: decreased *ADH* is released by the posterior pituitary gland. Remember this as **CIVIT**:
  - ○ **C**ongenital defect in *ADH* gene.
  - ○ **I**diopathic.
  - ○ **V**ascular.
  - ○ **I**nfection: meningoencephalitis.
  - ○ **T**umour (e.g. pituitary adenoma), **T**uberculosis and **T**rauma.
- Nephrogenic: the kidney does not respond to *ADH*. Remember this as **DIMC**:
  - ○ **D**rugs, e.g. lithium.
  - ○ **I**nherited.
  - ○ **M**etabolic ↓ potassium, ↑ calcium.
  - ○ **C**hronic renal disease.
  - (See also Figure 5.1)

Signs and symptoms

- Polydypsia.
- Polyuria.
- Dehydration.

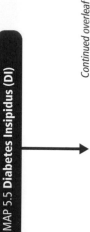

FIGURE 5.1 **Causes of Diabetes Insipidus**

Posterior pituitary gland → ADH → Kidney → H$_2$O reabsorption

1 Cranial cause   2 Nephrogenic cause

MAP 5.5 **Diabetes Insipidus (DI)**

Continued overleaf

Map 5.5 Diabetes Insipidus (DI)

The Endocrine System

Complications

- Electrolyte imbalance.
- Dehydration.

MAP 5.5 Diabetes Insipidus (DI) *(Continued)*

Treatment

This depends on the cause:

- Conservative: patient education. Education on how to monitor fluid levels and dietary salt levels. Advise patients to wear a MedicAlert® bracelet.
- Medical:

Cranial cause	Nephrogenic cause
Desmopressin – a synthetic replacement for vasopressin; it increases the number of aquaporin-2 channels in the distal convoluted tubules and the collecting ducts. This increases water reabsorption	High-dose desmopressin
	Correction of electrolyte imbalances
	Thiazide diuretics
	Prostaglandin synthase inhibitors

- Surgical: excision of tumour if indicated.

Investigations

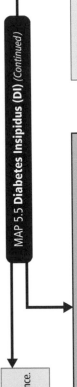

Investigation	Cranial cause	Nephrogenic cause
Plasma osmolality	↑	↑
Urine osmolality	↓	↓
Plasma Na$^+$	↑	↑
24-h urine volume	>2 L	>2 L
Water deprivation test	Urine does not concentrate	Urine does not concentrate
After treatment with desmopressin	Urine becomes concentrated	Urine does not concentrate
MRI	Look for abnormality of the pituitary gland, e.g. tumour	

HYPOPARATHYROIDISM

What is it?

This occurs when too little PTH is produced from the parathyroid gland. It may be categorised into congenital, acquired, transient and inherited causes.

Type	Cause
Congenital	DiGeorge's syndrome (chromosome 22q11.2 deletion)
Acquired	Complication of parathyroidectomy or thyroidectomy
Transient	Neonates born prematurely
Inherited	Pseudohypoparathyroidism Pseudopseudohypoparathyroidism

Signs and symptoms

These depend on the cause: abdominal pain, myalgia, muscle spasm, seizures, fatigue, headaches, carpopedal spasm, Chvostek's sign, Trousseau's sign.

Treatment

- Conservative: diet high in calcium and low in phosphate. Support for parents.
- Medical: calcium and vitamin D supplements.

Investigations

Investigation	Hypopara-thyroidism	Pseudohypo-parathyroidism	Pseudopseudo-hypoparathyroidism
PTH level	↓	↑	Normal
Serum calcium	↓	↓	Normal
Serum phosphate	↑	↑	Normal

Other investigations include:
- Bloods: FBC, U&Es, LFTs, creatinine, urea.
- ECG: arrhythmias.
- ECHO: cardiac structural defects (DiGeorge's syndrome).
- Radiology: X-ray of hand (pseudohypoparathyroidism patients have shorter 4th and 5th metacarpals).

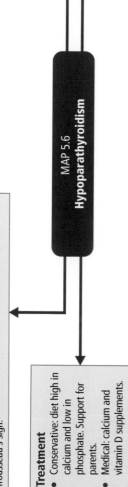

MAP 5.6
Hypoparathyroidism

Complications

- Renal calculi.
- Arrhythmias.
- Cataract formation.
- Dental problems.

Map 5.6 Hypoparathyroidism

Map 5.7 Hyperparathyroidism

HYPERPARATHYROIDISM

What is it?

This occurs when too much parathyroid hormone (PTH) is produced from the parathyroid gland. It may be categorised into primary, secondary and tertiary causes.

Causes

Type	Cause
Primary	Parathyroid adenoma Parathyroid hyperplasia Parathyroid carcinoma Drug induced, e.g. lithium
Secondary	Vitamin D deficiency Chronic kidney injury
Tertiary	Prolonged secondary hyperparathyroidism

Signs and symptoms

These depend on the cause.

Primary – *Bones, moans, groans and stones'*	Secondary
Asymptomatic Bones, e.g. pain, osteoporosis Moans, e.g. depression, fatigue Groans, e.g. myalgia Stones, e.g. kidney stones	Osteomalacia Rickets Renal osteodystrophy

Investigations

Investigation	Primary	Secondary	Tertiary
PTH level	↑	↑	↑
Serum calcium	↑	↓	↑
Serum phosphate	↓	↑	↓

Other investigations include:
- Bloods: FBC, U&Es, LFTs, creatinine.
- Urine calcium level.
- Dual energy X-ray (DEXA) scan.
- Radiology:
  - Ultrasound scan of kidneys and neck.
  - Plain X-ray (for bone changes).
  - Parathyroid gland biopsy.

MAP 5.7
Hyperparathyroidism

Treatment

Type of treatment	Primary	Secondary	Tertiary
Conservative	Monitoring Increase oral fluid intake	Diet low in phosphate and high in calcium	–
Medical	Bisphosphonates	Calcimimetics, e.g. cinacalcet	–
Surgical	Parathyroidectomy	Parathyroidectomy if unresponsive to medical therapy	Para-thyroidectomy

Complications
- Renal calculi.
- Acute pancreatitis.
- Peptic ulceration.
- Calcification of the cornea.

Map 5.7 Hyperparathyroidism

Map 5.8 Conn's Syndrome

Signs and symptoms

- Hypertension.
- Symptoms and signs associated with hypokalaemia; muscle weakness, muscle cramps, tetany, paraesthesia, cardiac arrythmias.
- Abdominal pain and ileus associated with hypokalaemia.

What is Conn's syndrome?

This is a condition of hyperaldosteronism. It is a rare cause of secondary hypertension.

Causes

The most common cause of Conn's syndrome is an adrenal adenoma. Other causes include hyperplasia of the zona glomerulosa or adrenal carcinoma.

Aldosterone is a mineralocorticoid that is released from the zona glomerulosa of the adrenal medulla. Aldosterone increases the absorption of Na^+ (and therefore water) in exchange for K^+ by stimulating the Na^+/K^+ pump present within the renal tubular epithelial cells within the distal convoluted tubule, the collecting tubules and the collecting ducts.

Therefore, with too much aldosterone as present in Conn's syndrome, there is increased blood pressure as a result of increased Na^+ and water absorption but also hypokalaemia.

MAP 5.8 **Conn's Syndrome**

Treatment

- Conservative: patient education, management of cardiovascular risk factors.
- Medical: treatment depends on the underlying cause but, generally, the aim of treatment is to normalise blood pressure, electrolytes and aldosterone levels. Bilateral adrenal hyperplasia is typically treated with potassium-sparing agents spironolactone or eplerenone.
- Surgical: adrenalectomy. Patient blood pressure needs to be optimised pre-operatively typically with spironolactone or eplerenone.

Investigations

- Blood tests as per the investigation of hypertension pathway according to NICE guidelines (see Mind Map 1.6): FBC, U&Es, LFTs, TFTs, lipid profile, cholesterol, HbA1c.
- Blood pressure monitoring.
- ECG.
- Conn's specific blood tests: these will reveal hypokalaemia, hypernatraemia and metabolic alkalosis.
  - ARR (aldosterone:renin ratio).
  - Radiology: CT abdomen to evaluate for adenoma.
  - Plasma 18-hydroxycorticosterone is elevated in adenoma.
  - +/– adrenal venous sampling if adenoma is very small and to confirm lateralisation; however, this is an invasive procedure and associated with complications.

Complications

- Related to prolonged, uncontrolled hypertension: cardiovascular disease, myocardial infarction, heart failure, stroke, retinopathy, renal disease.
- Related to hypokalaemia, including cardiac arrhythmias and death.

Map 5.9 Cushing's Syndrome

What is Cushing's syndrome?

This is a collection of signs and symptoms that occur when a patient has long-term exposure to cortisol. There are many causes of Cushing's syndrome and they may be classified as exogenous or endogenous causes.

Causes

Type	Cause
Exogenous	Iatrogenic, e.g. prescription of glucocorticoids for asthma
Endogenous	This may be split into adrenocorticotrophic hormone (ACTH) dependent and ACTH independent causes: • **ACTH dependent:** ○ Cushing's disease: this occurs when ACTH is produced from a pituitary adenoma. Use a low-dose dexamethasone test to confirm ○ Ectopic ACTH production (usually from small cell lung cancer) • **ACTH independent: CARS:** ○ **C**ancer: adrenal adenoma ○ **A**drenal nodular hyperplasia ○ **R**are causes: McCune–Albright syndrome ○ **S**teroid use

MAP 5.9 Cushing's Syndrome

Investigations

- Diagnostic tests: urinary free cortisol, low-dose and high-dose dexamethasone suppression test.
- Bloods: FBC, U&Es, LFTs, glucose, lipid levels.
- Radiology: CXR (look for lung cancer and vertebral collapse).
- Other: dual energy X-ray (DEXA) scan.

Signs and symptoms

- Moon face.
- Central obesity.
- Buffalo hump.
- Acne.
- Hypertension.
- Hyperglycaemia.
- Striae.
- Vertebral collapse.
- Proximal muscle wasting.
- Psychosis.

Treatment

- Conservative: education about the condition. Advise patient to decrease alcohol consumption since alcohol increases cortisol levels.
- Medical: ketoconazole, metyrapone, mitotane. Treat complications such as hypertension and diabetes mellitus.
- Surgical: trans-sphenoidal surgery to remove pituitary adenoma or bilateral adrenalectomy to remove adrenal adenoma, if indicated.

Complications

- Osteoporosis.
- Diabetes mellitus.
- Hypertension.
- Immunosuppression.
- Cataracts.
- Striae formation.
- Ulcers.

FIGURE 5.2 **The Hypothalamic–Pituitary–Adrenal Axis**

Pituitary gland → ACTH → Adrenal cortex → Cortisol

Destruction of the adrenal cortex leads to cortisol deficiency

Functions: 3As
1 **A** – m**A**ke glucose in the liver
2 **A** – **A**ntistress pathway
3 **A** – **A**nti-inflammatory pathway

Figure 5.2 The Hypothalamic–Pituitary–Adrenal Axis

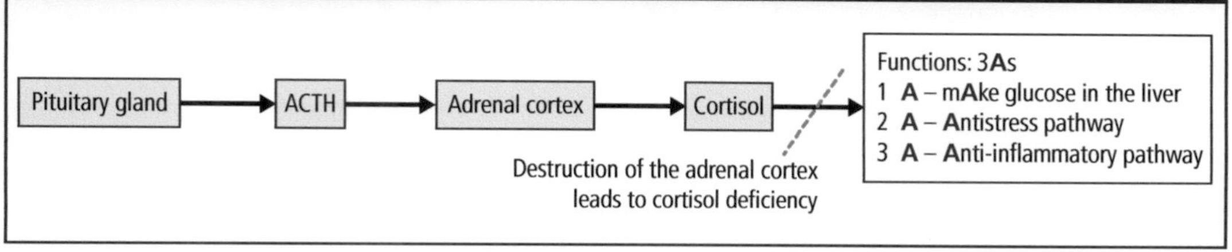

Map 5.10 Adrenal Insufficiency

What is adrenal insufficiency?

This occurs when the adrenal glands fail to produce sufficient steroid hormone. The causes of adrenal insufficiency may be categorised into primary and secondary adrenal failure.

Causes

Type	Cause
Primary	• Addison's disease; causes: **MAIL**: 　○ **M**etastases from breast, lung and renal cancers 　○ **A**utoimmune 　○ **I**nfections, e.g. tuberculosis (commonest cause) and opportunistic infections, such as cytomegalovirus (CMV) in HIV patients 　○ **L**ymphomas • Idiopathic • Postadrenalectomy
Secondary	• Prolonged prednisolone use • Pituitary adenoma • Sheehan's syndrome

Signs and symptoms

- Unintentional weight loss.
- Myalgia.
- Weakness.
- Fatigue.
- Postural hypotension.
- Abdominal pain.
- Skin pigmentation.
- Body hair loss.
- Diarrhoea.
- Nausea.
- Vomiting.
- Depression.

Investigations

- Diagnostic tests:
  - Adrenocorticotrophic hormone (ACTH) and cortisol measurements.
  - Insulin tolerance test.
  - Short tetracosactide test aka Short Synacthen test.
- Bloods: FBC, U&Es (↓ Na⁺, ↑ K⁺), LFTs, glucose, lipid levels, serum calcium.
- Radiology:
  - CXR (look for lung cancer).
  - CT and MRI scan of the adrenal glands.

Treatment

- Conservative: patient education. Patient must carry a steroid alert card.
- Medical: replace glucocorticoids and mineralocorticoids with hydrocortisone and fludrocortisone; treat complications.
- Surgery: surgical excision of tumour, if indicated.

MAP 5.10 **Adrenal Insufficiency**

FIGURE 5.3 Anatomy of the Adrenal Cortex and Adrenal Medulla

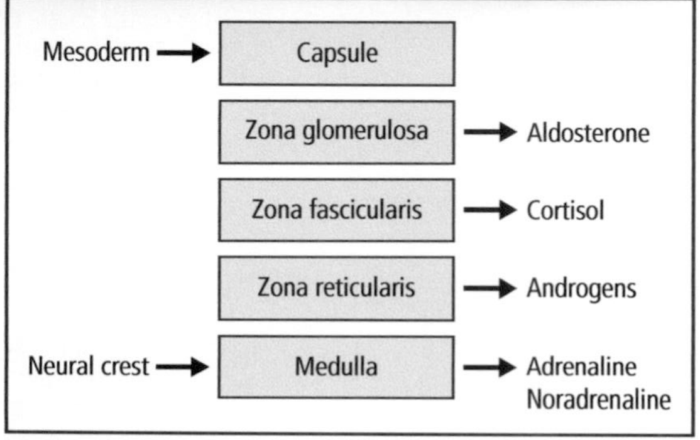

Mesoderm ➔

| Capsule |
Zona glomerulosa	➔ Aldosterone
Zona fascicularis	➔ Cortisol
Zona reticularis	➔ Androgens
Medulla	➔ Adrenaline / Noradrenaline

Neural crest ➔

Complications

- Adrenal crisis.
- Hyperkalaemia.
- Hypoglycaemia.
- Eosinophilia.
- Alopecia.
- Addison's disease is associated with other conditions such as **3PGH**:
  ○ **P**ernicious anaemia.
  ○ **P**rimary ovarian failure.
  ○ **P**olyglandular syndrome.
  ○ **G**raves' disease.
  ○ **H**ashimoto's thyroiditis.

Map 5.11 Acromegaly

What is acromegaly?

Acromegaly is a syndrome that results from excessive growth hormone (GH) production after fusion of the epiphyseal plates. Excess GH produced before epiphyseal plate fusion causes gigantism.

Causes

- Pituitary adenoma (most common).
- GH-releasing hormone (GHRH) production from bronchial carcinoid.

Signs and symptoms

- Increased jaw size.
- Increased hand size.
- Macroglossia.
- Lower pitch of voice.
- Carpal tunnel syndrome.
- Ask to see old photographs of the patient and note changes in appearance.

Investigations

- Bloods: FBC, U&Es, creatinine, LFTs, glucose, lipid levels, GH levels, glucose tolerance test, insulin-like growth factor (IGF)-1 levels (raised), prolactin levels.
- Radiology:
  ○ CXR.
  ○ CT and MRI scans.
- ECG and ECHO: assess for cardiac complications, e.g. cardiomyopathy.
- Visual field testing: bilateral hemianopia.

MAP 5.11 Acromegaly

Complications

- Increased risk of cardiovascular disease.
- Hypertension.
- Diabetes mellitus.
- Increased risk of colon cancer.
- Erectile dysfunction.
- Postsurgical, e.g. infection, cerebrospinal fluid (CSF) leak.
- Renal calculi (10%), as hypercalciuria may be induced by GH excess.
- Local pressure effects from pituitary adenoma, e.g. bitemporal hemianopia, headache.
- Increased risk of colonic polyps and uterine polyps.

Treatment

- Conservative: patient education. Inform the patient that bone changes will not revert after treatment.
- Medical:
  ○ Somatostatin analogues, e.g. octreotide.
  ○ Dopamine agonists, e.g. cabergoline.
  ○ GH receptor antagonists, e.g. pegvisomant.
- Surgery: trans-sphenoidal surgical excision of the adenoma is the treatment of choice.

Map 6.1 Regions of the Brain

Frontal lobe

- Is responsible for motor control of the opposite side of the body, e.g. the left frontal lobe has motor control of the right side of the body.
- Controls emotion and insight.
- The dominant hemisphere is responsible for speech output (Broca's area)
- Primary motor cortex: located in the posterior portion of the frontal lobe. This area plans and executes movement.
- Broca's area: located in the frontal lobe, just superior to the lateral fissure. It is responsible for the formation of speech.

Basal ganglia

- Is an interconnection of deep nuclei:
  o Putamen and globus pallidus: together they form the lentiform nucleus.
  o Caudate nucleus.
  o Substantia nigra.
  o Subthalamic nucleus.
- Integrates motor and sensory inputs.

Parietal lobe

- Is responsible for sensation of the opposite side of the body.
- It is also responsible for spatial awareness.
- Somatosensory cortex: located in the anterior cortex of the parietal lobe. It processes pain, pressure and touch.

MAP 6.1 Regions of the Brain

Cerebellum

This is split into 3 lobes:
1 The paleocerebellum: maintains gait.
2 The neocerebellum: maintains postural tone and is responsible for the coordination of fine motor skills.
3 The archicerebellum: maintains balance.

Occipital lobe

- Is responsible for vision.
- Primary visual cortex is located within this lobe.

Temporal lobe

- Is responsible for memory and emotion.
- In the dominant hemisphere it is responsible for the comprehension of speech (Wernicke's area).
- Wernicke's area: allows spoken and written language to be comprehended. It is located just posterior to the superior temporal gyrus.
- Primary auditory complex: responsible for hearing. It is located within the temporal lobe bilaterally.

FIGURE 6.1 **The Blood Supply of the Brain**

Circle of Willis

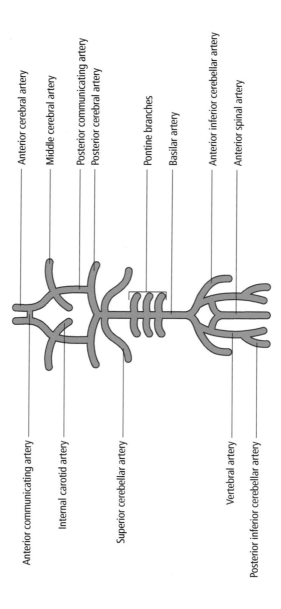

Anterior communicating artery

Internal carotid artery

Superior cerebellar artery

Posterior inferior cerebellar artery

Anterior cerebral artery

Middle cerebral artery

Posterior communicating artery

Posterior cerebral artery

Pontine branches

Basilar artery

Anterior inferior cerebellar artery

Anterior spinal artery

Vertebral artery

Figure 6.1 The Blood Supply of the Brain

Table 6.1 The Cranial Nerves and Their Lesions

TABLE 6.1 The Cranial Nerves and Their Lesions

Nerve	Sensory or motor	Location	Function	Lesion
I: Olfactory	Sensory	Cribriform plate of the ethmoid bone	Sense of smell	Loss of smell (anosmia)
II: Optic	Sensory	Optic canal	Sight	Different visual field losses depending on the location of the lesion
III: Oculomotor	Motor	Superior orbital fissure	Innervates the superior, medial and inferior rectus muscles as well as the levator palpebrae superioris, inferior oblique and sphincter pupillae	Eye moves down and out due to unopposed action of the superior oblique and lateral rectus muscles; ptosis (drooping eyelid) and mydriasis (dilated pupil) are observed
IV: Trochlear	Motor	Superior orbital fissure	Innervates the superior oblique muscle	Diplopia and eye moves down and in
V: Trigeminal	Motor and sensory	V1: ophthalmic nerve: superior orbital fissure V2: maxillary nerve: foramen rotundum V3: mandibular nerve: foramen ovale	Sensation of the face and innervates the muscles of mastication; test corneal reflex	Decreased facial sensation and jaw weakness
VI: Abducens	Motor	Superior orbital fissure	Innervates the lateral rectus muscle	Eye deviates medially

VII: **F**acial	Motor and sensory	Internal acoustic canal and exits through the stylomastoid foramen	Innervates the muscles of facial expression, stapedius, posterior belly of the digastric muscle, stylohyoid, taste anterior 2/3 of tongue, the lacrimal gland and the salivary glands (not parotids)	Upper motor neuron (UMN): asymmetry of lower face with forehead sparing Lower motor neuron (LMN): asymmetry of upper and lower face; loss of taste, hyperacusis and eye irritation due to ↓ lacrimation
VIII: **V**estibulocochlear	Sensory	Internal acoustic canal	Sense of sound and balance	Deafness and vertigo
IX: **G**lossopharyngeal	Motor and sensory	Jugular foramen	Supplies taste to posterior 1/3 of tongue and innervates the parotids as well as stylopharyngeus	Decreased gag reflex, uvular deviation away from lesion
X: **V**agus	Motor and sensory	Jugular foramen	Innervates laryngeal and pharyngeal muscles (not stylopharyngeus) and parasympathetic supply to thoracic and abdominal viscera	Dysphagia, recurrent laryngeal nerve palsies and pseudobulbar palsies
XI: spinal **A**ccessory	Motor	Jugular foramen	Innervates trapezius and sternocleidomastoid muscles	Patient cannot shrug and displays weak head movement
XII: **H**ypoglossal	Motor	Hypoglossal canal	Innervates the muscles of the tongue (except for the palatoglossal, which is supplied by the vagus nerve)	Tongue deviates towards the side of weakness during protrusion

Table 6.1 The Cranial Nerves and Their Lesions

Figure 6.2 Ascending and Descending Spinal Pathways

FIGURE 6.2 **Ascending and Descending Spinal Pathways**

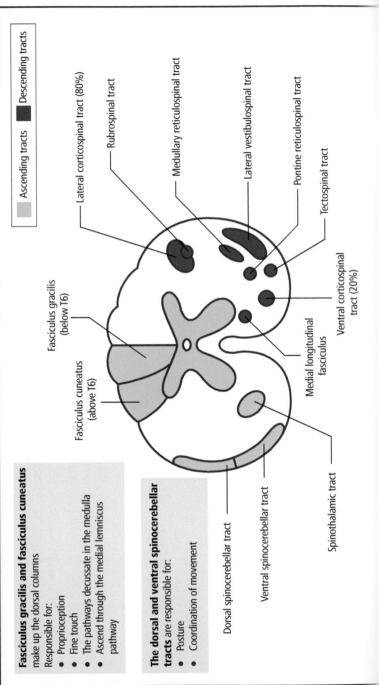

Ascending tracts   Descending tracts

Fasciculus gracilis and fasciculus cuneatus
make up the dorsal columns
Responsible for:
- Proprioception
- Fine touch
- The pathways decussate in the medulla
- Ascend through the medial lemniscus
  pathway

The dorsal and ventral spinocerebellar tracts are responsible for:
- Posture
- Coordination of movement

Lateral corticospinal tract (80%)

Rubrospinal tract

Medullary reticulospinal tract

Lateral vestibulospinal tract

Pontine reticulospinal tract

Tectospinal tract

Ventral corticospinal tract (20%)

Medial longitudinal fasciculus

Fasciculus gracilis (below T6)

Fasciculus cuneatus (above T6)

Dorsal spinocerebellar tract

Ventral spinocerebellar tract

Spinothalamic tract

Dorsal spinocerebellar tract
- Originates from Clarke's column
- Location: inferior cerebellar peduncle
- Ipsilateral

Ventral spinocerebellar tract
- Location: superior cerebellar peduncle
- Contralateral

Spinothalamic tract
- Decussate at level of entry
- Anterior: crude touch
- Posterior: pain and temperature

Responsible for:
- Pain
- Pressure
- Non-discriminative touch

Lateral corticospinal tract (80%)
- Voluntary skilled movements at the DISTAL parts of limbs

Tectospinal tract
- Originates in the superior colliculus

Responsible for:
- Reflective movements of the head in response to visual/auditory stimuli

Rubrospinal tract
- Location: red nucleus of the midbrain
- Afferent fibres are received from the cerebellum and motor cortex

Responsible for:
- Control of limb flexor muscles

Medullary reticulospinal tract
- Bilateral

Responsible for:
- Reflex activity
- Control of breathing
- Control of alpha and gamma neurons

Lateral vestibulospinal tract
- From vestibular nucleus in pons and medulla

Responsible for:
- EXTENSOR muscle tone
- Posture

Pontine reticulospinal tract
- Ipsilateral

Figure 6.2 Ascending and Descending Spinal Pathways

Map 6.2 Stroke

What is a stroke?

A stroke is a vascular insult to the brain causing a focal neurological deficit. This occurs due to ischaemic infarct or haemorrhage, which disrupts the blood supply to the brain.

Signs and symptoms

These vary depending on the circulation affected by the infarct or haemorrhage, e.g. new onset vertigo can be a sign of a posterior circulation stroke.

Acute signs and symptoms may be remembered as **FAST**:

- **Face**: unilateral drooping.
- **Arms**: these may feel weak and numb. Patient may not be able to lift them.
- **Speech**: slurring of speech.
- **Time**: time for emergency medical attention, call 999 (UK) immediately.

Stroke may also be associated with transient ischaemic attack (TIA). This is a focal neurological deficit where symptoms last <24 h due to temporary occlusion of the cerebral circulation. Patients may describe amaurosis fugax – loss of sight described as 'curtains descending'. The phenomenon lasts <24 h and is usually followed by a stroke within 90 days.

Risk factors

- ↑ Blood pressure.
- Atrial fibrillation (AF).
- Diabetes mellitus.
- Smoking.
- Alcohol.
- Previous stroke.
- The oral contraceptive pill.
- Disorder that increases clotting.
- Cocaine use.
- ↑ Cholesterol.

Investigations

- Bloods: FBC, U&Es, LFTs, PTT, glucose, cholesterol levels.
- Other: ECG for AF and ECHO for structural abnormalities. Glascow Coma Scale to assess level of consciousness.
- Radiology: CT head and diffusion-weighted MRI (DWI) immediately if any indication of stroke. It is important to distinguish between haemorrhagic and ischaemic stroke since treatment options differ.

Complications

- Hydrocephalus.
- Increased risk of deep vein thrombosis (DVT).
- Aphasia.
- Dysphagia.
- Decreased muscle movement.
- Amnesia.
- Depression.

MAP 6.2 **Stroke**

Causes

- Haemorrhagic causes:
  - Central nervous system bleeds from trauma.
  - Ruptured aneurysm.
- Ischaemic causes:
  - Small vessel occlusion.
  - Atherothromboembolism.
  - Cardiac emboli.
  - Emboli secondary to AF.

Treatment

- Conservative: patient and family education, initiate early mobilisation, commence stroke rehabilitation, assess speech and swallowing. Assess impact of activities of daily living (ADLs) using Barthel's index.
- Medical:
  - TIA patients:
    - Assess risk of subsequent stroke using ABCD[2] (high risk is a score >6, low risk is a score <4). ABCD[2]: **A**ge >60 years (1 point); **B**lood pressure >140/90 mmHg (1 point); **C**linical features: unilateral weakness (2 points), isolated speech disturbance (1 point); **D**uration of symptoms: >60 min (2 points), 10–59 min (1 point); **D**iabetes (1 point).
    - Start aspirin 300 mg.
  - Ischaemic stroke patients without haemorrhage:
    - Thrombolysis with alteplase within 3 h (patients >80 years) and within 4.5 h (patients <80 years).
    - Start aspirin 300 mg (unless contraindications).
    - These patients need to be discussed with the acute stroke team on call and the interventional neuroradiologist re. management.
  - Haemorrhagic stroke patients:
    - Prothrombin complex concentrate.
    - Intravenous vitamin K.
    - To be discussed with acute stroke team on call +/– interventional neuroradiologist.
- Surgical:
  - Referral for acute intracerebral haemorrhage.
  - Referral for decompressive hemicraniectomy.

TABLE 6.2 Dementia

This is a syndrome of a progressive global decline in cognitive function

Type of dementia	Causes	Signs and symptoms	Investigations	Treatment	Complications

Alzheimer's disease	Exact cause unknown
	
	Risk factors include:
	• Down's syndrome due to ↑*APP* gene load
	• Familial gene associations:
	  ○ Amyloid precursor protein (APP): chromosome 21
	  ○ Presenilin-1: chromosome 14
	  ○ Presenilin-2: chromosome 1
	  ○ Apolipoprotein E4 (ApoE4) alleles: chromosome 19
	• Hypothyroidism
	• Previous head trauma
	• Family history of Alzheimer's disease
		Amnesia
		Disorientation
		Changes in personality
		Decreasing self care
		Apraxia
		Agnosia
		Aphasia
		Lexical anomia
		Paranoid delusions
		Depression
		Wandering
		Aggression
		Sexual disinhibition
			Mental state examination
			Addenbrooke's Cognitive Examination (ACE-III)
			Bloods: FBC, U&Es, LFTs, TFTs, CRP, ESR, glucose, calcium, magnesium, phosphate, VDRL, HIV serology, vitamin B_{12} and folate levels, blood culture, ECG, lumbar puncture, CXR, CT scan, MRI scan, SPECT
			3 main findings on histology:
			BAT:
			• **B**eta-amyloid plaques
			• ↓ **A**cetylcholine
			• neurofibrillary **T**angles
				Memantine: inhibits glutamate by blocking N-methyl-D-aspartate (NMDA) receptors
				Donepezil: acetylcholinesterase inhibitor
				Rivastigmine: acetylcholinesterase inhibitor
					Amnesia
					Increased risk of infection
					Dysphagia
					Urinary incontinence
					Increased risk of falls

Vascular dementia	Is the second most common cause of dementia It is caused by infarcts of small and medium-sized vessels in the brain	It follows a deteriorating stepwise progression. There are 3 types: 1 Vascular dementia following stroke	Mental state examination ACE-III Bloods: FBC, U&Es, LFTs, TFTs, CRP, ESR, glucose, calcium, magnesium, phosphate, VDRL,	Dietary advice Smoking cessation Treat diabetes mellitus and hypertension Aspirin	Significant comorbidity, e.g. cardiovascular disease and renal disease

Table 6.2 Dementia

			Neuroleptic hypersensitivity Autonomic dysfunction Fluctuating blood pressure Arrhythmias Urinary incontinence Dysphagia Increased risk of falls
	Genetic association with cerebral autosomal dominant arteriopathy (CADASIL) with subcortical infarcts and leuco-encephalopathy on chromosome 19	2 Multi-infarct dementia following multiple strokes 3 Binswanger's disease following microvascular infarcts Amnesia Disorientation Changes in personality Decreasing self care Depression Signs of upper motor neuron (UMN) lesions, e.g. brisk reflexes Seizures	HIV serology, vitamin B_{12} and folate levels, cholesterol levels, vasculitis screen, syphilis serology ECG, lumbar puncture, CXR, CT scan, MRI scan, SPECT
Dementia with Lewy bodies	Associated with Parkinson's disease Avoid antipsychotic drugs in these patients	Is a triad of: 1 Parkinsonism: bradykinesia, gait disorder 2 Hallucinations: predominantly visual hallucinations, usually of animals and people 3 Disease process follows a fluctuating course	Mental state examination ACE-III CT scan, MRI scan, SPECT scan ApoE genotype Lewy bodies, ubiquitin proteins and alpha-synuclein found on histology	AVOID ANTIPSYCHOTICS: causes hypersensitivity to neuroleptics Levodopa may be used to treat Parkinson's symptoms but these may worsen psychotic symptoms

Continued overleaf

Table 6.2 Dementia

TABLE 6.2 **Dementia** (*Continued*)

This is a syndrome of a progressive global decline in cognitive function

Type of dementia	Causes	Signs and symptoms	Investigations	Treatment	Complications
Frontotemporal dementia (Pick's disease)	Involved genes are those coding for tau protein located on chromosome 17q21.32 and granulin on chromosome 17q21.32, and hexanucleotide repeat expansion of the chromosome 9 open-reading-frame 72 (C9orf72) on chromosomal location 9p21.2	Amnesia Disorientation Changes in personality Decreasing self-care Mutism Echolalia Overeating Parkinsonism Disinhibition	Mental state examination ACE-III CT scan, MRI scan, SPECT scan Histology – depends on subtype: • Microvacuolar type: microvacuolation • Pick type: widespread gliosis, no microvacuolation • Motor neuron disease (MND) type: histological changes like MND	Currently none. Only supportive treatment available	Increased risk of falls Increased risk of infection
Huntington's dementia	A complication of Huntington's disease (see page 238), which is an autosomal dominant disorder in which there is a defective gene on chromosome 4 Causes uncontrollable choreiform movements and dementia	Uncontrollable choreiform movements Depression Irritability Anxiety Psychosis Obsessive–compulsive behaviour	Diagnostic genetic testing	No cure. Treat symptoms: • Chorea: an atypical antipsychotic agent • Obsessive–compulsive thoughts and irritability: selective serotonin reuptake inhibitors (SSRIs)	Dysphagia Increased risk of falls Increased risk of infection

Table 6.2 Dementia

Creutzfeldt–Jakob disease (CJD)	Caused by prions Progressive and without cure There is also variant CJD (vCJD), which has an earlier onset of death	Rapidly progressive dementia (4–5 months) Amnesia Disorientation Changes in personality Depression Psychosis Ataxia Seizures	EEG: triphasic spikes seen Lumbar puncture (LP): for 14-3-3 protein CT scan MRI scan	No cure	Increased risk of infection Coma Heart failure Respiratory failure
Other causes	HIV Vitamin B_{12} deficiency Syphilis Wilson's disease: autosomal recessive condition where copper accumulates within the tissues Dementia pugilistica: seen in boxers and patients who suffer multiple concussions; also known as 'punch-drunk' syndrome				

Table 6.2 Dementia

Map 6.3   Epilepsy

What is epilepsy?

This is a condition in which the brain is affected by recurrent seizures. These seizures may be defined in many different ways:

- Partial seizures: these are seizures that occur in one discrete part of the brain. These seizures may be simple (without alteration in consciousness) or complex (with alteration in consciousness).
- Generalised seizures: these seizures affect the brain globally. Consciousness is always altered. Examples include:
  - Absence seizures: often picked up in children who 'stare into space'. The seizure usually only lasts seconds.
  - Tonic–clonic seizures: involves convulsions and muscle rigidity. Usually last minutes.
  - Atonic seizures: involves a loss of muscle tone.
  - Myotonic: involves jerky muscle movements.
  - Secondary generalised: this is a generalised seizure that originates from a partial seizure.

Investigations

- Bloods: FBC, U&Es, LFTs, CRP, ESR, glucose, calcium levels.
- Radiology: CT scan, MRI scan.
- Other: ECG, LP, EEG.

Signs and symptoms

These depend on the region of the brain affected.

- Frontal lobe, remember **JAM**:
  - **J**acksonian march.
  - p**A**lsy (postictal Todd's palsy).
  - **M**otor features.
- Temporal lobe, remember **ADD FAT**:
  - **A**ura that the epileptic attack will occur.
  - **D**éjà-vu.
  - **D**elusional behaviour.
  - **F**ear/panic: hippocampal involvement.
  - **A**utomatisms.
  - **T**aste/smell: uncal involvement.
- Parietal and occipital lobe: visual and sensory disturbances.
- Others include: partial or generalised seizure with or without convulsions, tongue biting, migraines and depression.

MAP 6.3 **Epilepsy**

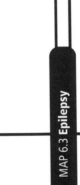

Causes

Seizures are caused by abnormal paroxysmal neuronal discharges in the brain, which are usually a result of some form of traumatic brain injury. These discharges display hypersynchronisation. The causes of epilepsy may be broadly classified into 3 types:

1 Idiopathic: cause for epilepsy is unknown.
2 Cryptogenic: cause for epilepsy is unknown, but there are signs suggesting it may be linked to brain injury, e.g. patient has autism or learning difficulties.
3 Symptomatic: cause known. Some causes of symptomatic epilepsy include:

VINDICATE:

○ Vascular: history of stroke.
○ Infection: history of meningitis or malaria.
○ Neoplasms: brain tumour.
○ Drugs: alcohol and illicit drug use.
○ Iatrogenic: drug withdrawal.
○ Congenital: family history of epilepsy.
○ Autoimmune: vasculitis.
○ Trauma: history of brain injury.
○ Endocrine: ↓ Na⁺, ↓ Ca²⁺, ↓ or ↑ glucose.

Complications

- Injuries whilst having seizure.
- Depression.
- Anxiety.
- Brain damage.
- Sudden unexplained death in epilepsy (SUDEP).

Treatment

- Conservative: patient and family education. Inform DVLA (UK).
- Medical: anticonvulsant therapy, see Table 6.3.
- Surgical: anterior temporal lobe resection, corpus callosotomy, tumour removal.

Map 6.3 Epilepsy

Table 6.3 Anticonvulsant Drugs

TABLE 6.3 Anticonvulsant Drugs

N.B. for a full description of epilepsy management and which drugs to use as first line, please follow the website link provided for NICE guidelines (Appendix Two)

Anticonvulsant agent	Mechanism of action	Uses	Side effects	Contraindications	Drug interactions
Carbamazepine	Blocks voltage-dependent Na$^+$ channels	All seizures except absence seizures Neuropathic pain, e.g. trigeminal neuralgia Bipolar disorder	Rash Sedation Drowsiness Hyponatraemia Dry mouth Blurring of vision Neutropenia Hallucinations	Pregnancy (it is teratogenic) Past history of bone marrow depression Acute porphyria	Alters metabolism of oral contraceptive pill Alters metabolism of warfarin Alters metabolism of corticosteroids
Phenytoin	Blocks voltage-dependent Na$^+$ channels	All seizures except pure absence seizures Seizure prevention post neurosurgery Trigeminal neuralgia Arrhythmia Digoxin toxicity	Rash Hypersensitivity reactions Ataxia Megaloblastic anaemia Hirsutism Gum hypertrophy Purple glove syndrome	Pregnancy (it is teratogenic) Sinus bradycardia Stokes–Adams syndrome Sinoatrial block Second-degree heart block Third-degree heart block	Sodium valproate alters (increases or decreases) phenytoin concentration Phenytoin increases metabolism of drugs like anticoagulants by enzyme induction Phenytoin reduces concentration of mirtazapine N.B. This drug has a narrow therapeutic index

Sodium valproate	Blocks voltage-dependent Na$^+$ channels Weakly inhibits gamma-aminobutyric acid (GABA) transaminase	All seizures Anxiety disorders Anorexia nervosa Bipolar disorder	Nausea Vomiting Weight gain Hair loss Thinning of hair Curling of hair Hepatotoxicity Tremor Parkinsonism Thrombocytopenia Encephalopathy	Pregnancy (it is teratogenic) Hepatic failure History of mitochondrial disease	Aspirin increases levels of sodium valproate Sodium valproate may enhance effects of anticoagulant coumarins Carbamazepine decreases levels of sodium valproate
Ethosuximide	Inhibits T-type Ca^{2+} channels	Absence seizures (used more frequently in children)	Nausea Vomiting Anorexia Hypersensitivity reactions Blood dyscrasias Ataxia	Pregnancy (it is teratogenic) Hepatic failure Affective disorders Systemic lupus erythematosus	Metabolism is inhibited by isoniazid Sodium valproate increases the level of ethosuximide Phenytoin and carbamazepine decrease the level of ethosuximide
Phenobarbital	Acts on GABA$_A$ receptors, enhancing synaptic inhibition	All seizures except absence seizures Status epilepticus (third line) Anaesthesia Neonatal seizures Cyclical vomiting syndrome Crigler–Najjar syndrome Gilbert's syndrome	Rash Sedation Depression Ataxia Amelogenesis imperfecta	Pregnancy (it is teratogenic) History of porphyria	Phenobarbital increases metabolism of coumarins Carbamazepine increases concentration of phenobarbital Phenobarbital decreases levels of itraconazole

Continued overleaf

Table 6.3 Anticonvulsant Drugs

TABLE 6.3 **Anticonvulsant Drugs** (*Continued*)

N.B. for a full description of epilepsy management and which drugs to use as first line, please follow the website link provided for NICE guidelines (Appendix Two)

Anticonvulsant agent	Mechanism of action	Uses	Side effects	Contraindications	Drug interactions
Benzodiazepines	Allosterically modifies GABA$_A$ receptor, thereby increasing Cl$^-$ conductance	Lorazepam used to treat status epilepticus (first line) Anxiety disorders Insomnia Seizures Alcohol withdrawal	Sedation Withdrawal syndrome Respiratory depression	Chronic obstructive pulmonary disease Sleep apnoea Myasthenia gravis Severe depression (increased suicidal tendencies)	Use cautiously with other central nervous system depressants, e.g. opioids and barbiturates Increasing sedative effect when used with antihistamines Increasing sedative effect when used with antipsychotics
Vigabatrin	Inhibits GABA transaminase	All seizures Seizures in patients who are resistant to other anticonvulsant medication	Sedation Headache Peripheral visual field defect Depression Psychosis Hallucinations	Hypersensitivity	Vigabatrin increases clearance of carbamazepine Vigabatrin decreases levels of phenytoin

Table 6.3 Anticonvulsant Drugs

Lamotrigine	Blocks voltage-dependent Na$^+$ channels Inhibits L-, N- and P-type Ca^{2+} channels	All seizures Bipolar disorder Severe depression Neuropathic pain, e.g. trigeminal neuralgia	Stevens–Johnson syndrome Toxic epidermal necrolysis (Lyell's syndrome) Rashes Nausea Ataxia	Hypersensitivity Hepatic failure	The oral contraceptive pill decreases levels of lamotrigine Carbemazepine decreases lamotrigine levels Rifampicin decreases levels of lamotrigine Valproate increases levels of lamotrigine
Gabapentin and pregabalin	Gapapentin is a GABA analogue Pregabalin is an analogue of gabapentin	All seizures Neuropathic pain Bipolar disorder	Sedation Ataxia	Hypersensitivity	When used with propoxyphene patients are more at risk of side effects such as dizziness and confusion Bioavailability of gabapentin increased by morphine

Table 6.3 Anticonvulsant Drugs

MAP 6.4 Multiple Sclerosis (MS)

What is MS?

This is thought to be a progressive autoimmune condition in which the neurons of the central nervous system demyelinate. Its progression may be classified into 4 subtypes:

1 Relapsing–remitting.
2 Primary progressive.
3 Secondary progressive.
4 Benign.

Causes

The exact cause of MS is not known but there are several factors that are thought to contribute:

- It is thought to be a type IV T cell-mediated immune response.
- Location: those who live further from the equator and Sardinians are at greater risk than other populations.
- Viruses may play a role, e.g. Epstein–Barr virus (EBV).
- Smoking is a risk factor.

Pathophysiology

- Plaques of demyelination, disseminated in time and space, interfere with neuronal transmission.
- Often patients enter remission but then relapse. This is because the demyelinated neurons do not heal fully.

Signs and symptoms

- Usually monosymptomatic.
- Symptoms relate to the location where plaques of demyelination occur. Remember these as **DOTS**:
  - **D**iplopia, **D**ysaesthesia.
  - **O**ptic neuritis: this is often a presenting symptom and patients complain of double vision (diplopia).
  - **T**rigeminal neuralgia, **T**runk and limb ataxia.
  - ↓ **S**ense of vibration.
- Uhthoff's phenomenon: symptoms worsen in hot conditions.

MAP 6.4 **Multiple Sclerosis (MS)**

Complications

- Urinary incontinence.
- Bowel incontinence.
- Depression.
- Epilepsy.
- Paralysis.

Treatment

- Conservative: patient education. Use diagnostic McDonald criteria and regularly assess ADLs as well as psychosocial impact of disease.
- Medical:
  - Interferon.
  - Methylprednisolone, a corticosteroid.
  - Glatiramer acetate, an immunomodulator.
  - Natalizumab, a monoclonal antibody.
  - Alemtuzumab, a monoclonal antibody.
  - Azathioprine, a purine analogue (immunosuppressant).
  - Mitoxantrone, a doxorubicin analogue.

Investigations

- LP: some proteins are altered in MS, e.g. oligoclonal bands.
- MRI scan: shows regions affected by inflammation and scarring, e.g. Dawson's fingers.

There is no specific blood test for MS but it is important to exclude other differentials in the work-up for this condition.

- Blood tests (FBC, U&Es, LFTs, CRP, vitamin B_{12}, folate and vitamin D, thyroid function tests, lipid panel), viral serology (anti-HIV, anti-HCV, HbsAg, anti-Hbs), VDRL-RPR, ANA (1/320 titre and patterns). If ANA positive, ENA profile, antiphospholipid antibodies, anti-ds DNA.
- MRI (cranial, cervical and thoracal).
- CSF analyses (CSF protein, CSF and concurrent blood glucose, CSF albumin and IgG, CSF lactate, serum albumin and IgG, CSF IgG index, CSF oligoclonal band analysis with IEF electrophoresis).
- In patients with optic neuritis: VEP and optic coherence tomography.
- Consider urodynamic studies.
- Consider cognitive testing.

McDonald criteria

McDonald diagnostic criteria for multiple sclerosis are clinical, radiographic and laboratory criteria used in the diagnosis of multiple sclerosis:

The criteria are:

- ≥2 clinical attacks.
  - With ≥2 lesions with objective clinical evidence.
    - With no additional data needed.
- ≥2 clinical attacks.
  - With 1 lesion with objective clinical evidence and clinical history suggestive of a previous lesion.
    - With no additional data needed.
- ≥2 clinical attacks.
  - With 1 lesion with objective clinical evidence and no clinical history suggestive of a previous lesion.
    - With dissemination in space evident on MRI.
- 1 clinical attack (i.e. clinically isolated syndrome).
  - With ≥2 lesions with objective clinical evidence.
    - With dissemination in time evident on MRI or demonstration of CSF-specific oligoclonal bands.
- 1 clinical attack (i.e. clinically isolated syndrome).
  - With 1 lesion with objective clinical evidence.
    - With dissemination in space evident on MRI.
    - With dissemination in time evident on MRI or demonstration of CSF-specific oligoclonal bands.

MAP 6.4 Multiple Sclerosis (MS)

Map 6.5 Parkinson's Disease

What is Parkinson's disease?

This is a progressive disorder of the central nervous system, which is due to dopamine depletion.

Causes

The exact cause of this degenerative disease is unknown but some postulated risk factors include:

- Male gender.
- Genetic component.
- Environmental exposure to insecticides, pesticides and herbicides.

Pathophysiology

- ↓ Dopamine producing cells in the pars compacta region of the substantia nigra, located in the midbrain.
- Dopamine produced is secreted to the putamen and caudate nucleus.
- ↑ Lewy bodies in the substantia nigra.

Signs and symptoms

Remember Facial TRAPS:

- **Facial**: expressionless face.
- Tremor (pill rolling tremor).
- Rigidity (cogwheel rigidity).
- Akinesia.
- Posture (stooped).
- Shuffling gait.

MAP 6.5 Parkinson's Disease

Investigations

There is no specific test for Parkinson's disease. It is a clinical diagnosis.

- CT scan and MRI scan may be arranged but these are usually normal.
- PET, SPECT and ioflupane (DaTSCAN) may measure basal ganglia dopaminergic function.

Treatment

- Conservative: patient education. Rehabilitation to improve gait and mobility. Regular assessment of activities of daily living.
- Medical:
  ○ Levodopa: crosses the blood–brain barrier (BBB) where it is converted to dopamine.
  ○ Carbidopa: always given with levodopa. It is a dopa decarboxylase inhibitor and prevents levodopa from being metabolised to dopamine in other regions of the body. Therefore, it acts to decrease peripheral side effects.
  ○ Selegiline: inhibits monoamine oxidase B (MAO-B). This enzyme breaks down dopamine.
  ○ Amantadine: dopamine agonist. Decreases Parkinsonian symptoms.
  ○ Surgical: this option is unlikely since drug regimens have improved.

Complications

- Dysphagia.
- Dementia.
- Increased risk of falls.
- Erectile dysfunction.

Figure 7.1 Components of a Full Blood Count

FIGURE 7.1 **Components of a Full Blood Count**

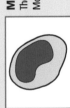

Monocytes

These are the precursors of tissue macrophages and dendritic antigen-presenting cells. They are phagocytic. Monocytosis may be associated with viral or chronic bacterial infections.

Lymphocytes

There are 3 key types of lymphocyte: T cells which are involved with cell-mediated immunity and cytotoxic adaptive immunity; B cells which are involved with humoral, adaptive immunity; and natural killer (NK) cells which play a role in cytotoxic innate immunity. Lymphocytosis may be seen in viral infections particularly EBV or CMV. Malignant proliferation of lymphocytes is seen in leukaemias and lymphomas.

Neutrophils

The most abundant granulocyte and part of the innate immune system. Neutrophils are the hallmark of acute inflammation. Neutrophilia is commonly seen as inflammation, bacterial infections, tissue necrosis and myeloproliferative disorders. Neutropenia may occur in viral infections.

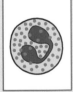

Eosinophils

This is a type of granulocyte that is typically associated with combating parasitic infections, allergy and asthma reactions. Eosinophilia may occur with parasitic infection, allergy disorders, skin disorders such as eczema, respiratory illnesses such as asthma and hypereosinophilic syndrome.

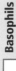

Basophils

The least common but largest granulocyte. Basophils have granules that contain heparin, histamine, proteoglycans and serotonin that play a role in coordinating the immune response. Basophilia is associated with myeloproliferative disorders.

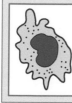

Macrophages

These are large phagocytes that engage in phagocytosis, i.e. engulfing and digesting microbes/foreign material, and move via an amoeboid process. There are 2 different types of macrophage. M1 macrophages promote the inflammatory process whereas M2 macrophages have an important anti-inflammatory role and release cytokines to facilitate this.

Erythrocytes (red blood cells)

These are characteristic in their biconcave disc appearance and absent nucleus. They have a lifespan of approximately 100–120 days and are packed with haemoglobin. They are responsible for the delivery of oxygen to the body's tissues. Erythropoiesis is the process by which new erythrocytes are made. This process takes about 7 days. Diseases involving red blood cells include anaemias, haemolysis (of any cause) and polycythaemias.

Platelets

These are fragments of cytoplasm from the megakaryocytes of bone marrow. They have no nucleus and are responsible for initiating blood clot development. Thrombocytopenia may be caused by bone marrow failure (e.g. bone marrow infiltration/side effects of certain drugs) or excessive consumption/destruction of platelets (e.g. dissemination intravascular coagulation).

Figure 7.1 Components of a Full Blood Count

MAP 7.1 Anaemia

What is anaemia?

Anaemia occurs when the haemoglobin (Hb) concentration is low.
This condition may be classified as microcytic, macrocytic or normocytic.

TABLE 7.1 Anaemia

Type of anaemia	Causes	Symptoms	Signs	Investigations	Treatment	Complications
Microcytic	Iron deficiency of varying cause, e.g. • Menorrhagia • Pregnancy • Gastrointestinal tract malignancy • Oesophagitis • Gastro-oesophageal reflux disease • Coeliac disease • Hookworm • Schistosomiasis • Diet low in iron Thalassaemia: see page 138	Fatigue Palpitations Headache Dyspnoea	Pallor Nail changes, e.g. koilonychia Angular cheilitis Atrophic glossitis	FBC • Microcytic, hypochromic anaemia • ↓ MCV (<80 fL) • ↓ MCH • ↓ Ferritin • ↓ Iron • ↑ Total iron binding capacity (TIBC) Blood film: anisocytosis and poikilocytosis Investigate causes, e.g. endoscopy, stool microscopy, barium enema	Treat cause Ferrous sulphate	Fatigue Increased risk of infection Heart failure
Macrocytic	Remember these as **FAT RBC:** **F**olate deficiency **A**lcohol **T**hyroid (hypothyroidism)	Fatigue Palpitations Headache Dyspnoea Irritability Depression	Pallor Glossitis Angular cheilitis Paraesthesiae Subacute degeneration of the spinal cord	FBC • ↓ Hb • ↑ MCV (>96 fL) • ↓ Vitamin B_{12} • ↓ Folate • ↓ Reticulocytes • ↓ Platelets (if severe)	Treat cause If pernicious anaemia then treat with hydroxocobalamin injections	Fatigue Heart failure Splenomegaly Neuropsychiatric and neurological complications

Map 7.1 Anaemia

	Causes	Symptoms	Signs	FBC	Treatment	Complications
	Reticulocytosis **B**$_{12}$ (vitamin B$_{12}$ deficiency)/ pernicious anaemia **Cytotoxic drugs**			• ↓WCC (if severe) Blood film: hypersegmented polymorphs (folate and vitamin B$_{12}$ deficiency); target cells observed in liver disease		Fatigue Heart failure
Normocytic	Haemolytic anaemia of varying cause, e.g. • Glucose-6-phosphate dehydrogenase deficiency • Hereditary spherocytosis • Erythroblastosis fetalis • Sickle cell disease • Warm antibody autoimmune haemolytic anaemia and cold agglutinin disease • Anaemia of chronic disease, e.g. rheumatoid arthritis • Aplastic anaemia	Fatigue Palpitations Headache Dyspnoea Symptoms of underlying disease	Pallor Signs of underlying disease	FBC • ↓ Hb • Normal MCV • Normal or ↑ ferritin	Treat cause	

Table 7.1 Anaemia

Map 7.2 Haemolytic Anaemia

What is haemolytic anaemia?

This is an anaemia that is caused by the breakdown of erythrocytes.

Causes

The causes of haemolytic anaemia may be inherited or acquired, and these are summarised in the following table.

Cause	Mechanism by which anaemia occurs		Examples
Inherited	Erythrocyte membrane defect		Hereditary spherocytosis
	Haemoglobin abnormalities		Sickle cell disease
			Thalassaemia
	Metabolic defects		Pyruvate kinase deficiency
			Glucose-6-phosphate dehydrogenase deficiency
Acquired	Immune		
		Autoimmune	Warm or cold autoimmune disease
		Alloimmune	Haemolytic transfusion reaction
	Non-immune		
		Membrane	Paroxysmal nocturnal haemoglobinuria
		Mechanical	Replacement cardiac valves
		Systemic	Secondary to renal disease/infections (malaria)/burns
		Iatrogenic	Drugs

Signs and symptoms

Depend on the underlying cause. Some may include:
- Pallor to skin and conjunctiva.
- Dark-coloured urine.
- Jaundice.
- Fever.
- Weakness and fatigue.
- Dizziness.
- Shortness of breath.
- Decreased exercise tolerance.
- Confusion.
- Splenomegaly.

MAP 7.2 **Haemolytic Anaemia**

Investigations

- Blood tests: FBC, U&Es, LFTs, Coag, iron studies.
- Peripheral blood smear.
- Diagnosis flow chart (Figure 7.2).

Initial laboratory tests for haemolysis

Test	Finding in haemolysis	Cause
Haptoglobin	Decreased	Binds free haemoglobin
Lactate dehydrogenase	Elevated	Released from lysis of red blood cells
Peripheral blood smear	Abnormal red blood cells	Based on cause of anaemia
Reticulocyte count	Increased	Marrow response to anaemia
Unconjugated bilirubin	Increased	Increased haemoglobin breakdown
Lactate urinalysis	Elevated	Free haemoglobin and its metabolites

Treatment

- Depends on the underlying cause.

Complications

- Gallstones, folate deficiency, parvovirus infections.

Map 7.2 Haemolytic Anaemia

Figure 7.2 Diagnosis of Haemolytic Anaemia

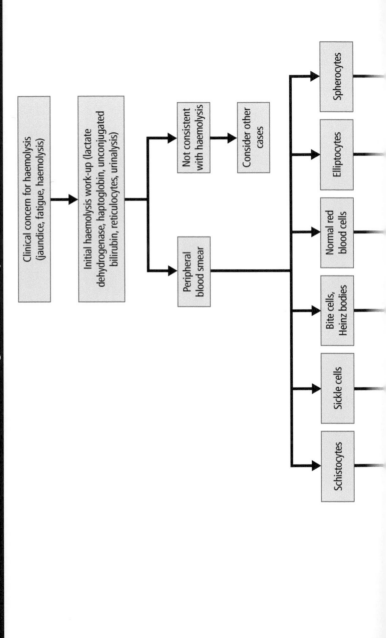

FIGURE 7.2 **Diagnosis of Haemolytic Anaemia**

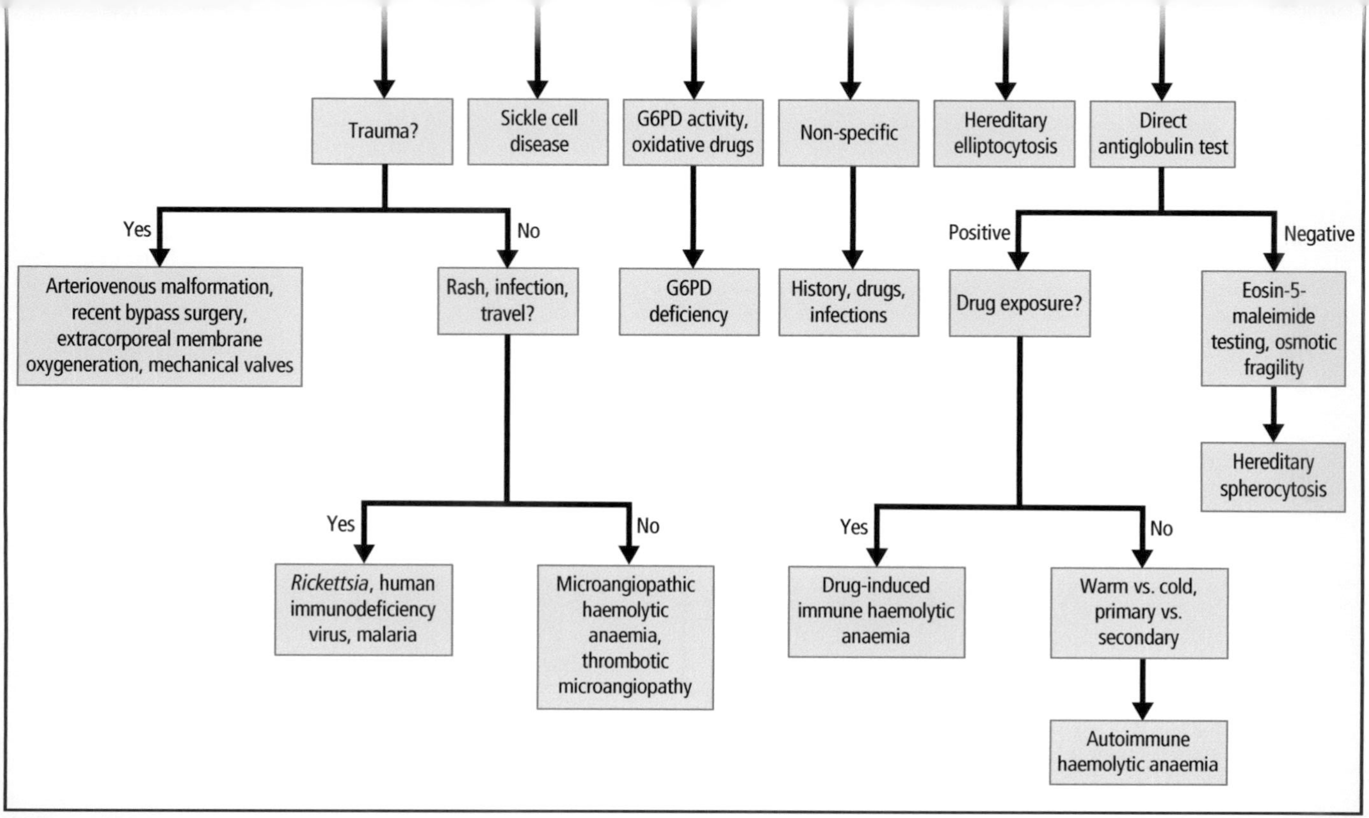

Figure 7.2 Diagnosis of Haemolytic Anaemia

Map 7.3   Hereditary Spherocytosis

What is hereditary spherocytosis?

This is an autosomal dominant condition in which the red blood cells are sphere shaped rather than biconcave. The different shape of the red blood cells means that these cells are more prone to haemolysis. It is the most common cause of inherited haemolytic anaemia.

Cause

Defects in the genes that code for certain red blood cell structural proteins e.g. spectrin, ankyrin, band 3 protein, etc. These genes are ANK1, SLC4A1, SPTA1, SPTB and EPB42.

Investigations

- Blood tests: FBC, U&Es, LFTs, Coag, iron studies. The eosin-5'-maleimide (EMA) binding test is the most accurate screen for hereditary sphero-cytosis (HS). The EMA binding test looks for the membrane proteins involved in HS. If these proteins are missing, the result suggests HS.
- Peripheral blood smear.
- Osmotic fragility tests.
- USS – to assess for gallstones.

Treatment

- Conservative: patient information, vaccinations, post-splenectomy vaccinations.
- Medical: folate supplementation, blood transfusions may be required for patients with severe disease.
- Surgical: splenectomy +/– cholecystectomy. If possible, splenectomy should be delayed until age 6 or older.

Complications

- Gallstones.
- Folate deficiency.
- Parvovirus infections.
- Post-splenectomy-related complications including OPSI and infections from opportunistic encapsulated organisms S. pneumoniae, H. influenzae and N. meningitidis.

MAP 7.3 **Hereditary Spherocytosis**

Signs and symptoms

These depend on the underlying cause. Some may include:

- Pallor to skin and conjunctiva.
- Dark-coloured urine.
- Jaundice.
- Fever.
- Weakness and fatigue.
- Dizziness.
- Shortness of breath.
- Decreased exercise tolerance.
- Confusion.
- Splenomegaly.

What is pernicious anaemia?

This is an autoimmune condition which results in decreased absorption of vitamin B_{12} and thus causes a megaloblastic anaemia.

Cause

Parietal cells present in the stomach produce intrinsic factor. Intrinsic factor binds to vitamin B_{12} and allows it to be absorbed in the terminal ileum. Some patients with pernicious anaemia have antibodies to parietal cells. Other patients have antibodies to intrinsic factor. These antibodies may be blocking or binding. Blocking antibodies bind to the intrinsic factor and block the binding of intrinsic factor and vitamin B_{12}. Binding antibodies bind to the already formed intrinsic factor and vitamin B_{12} complex, therefore preventing its absorption in the terminal ileum.

Signs and symptoms

The symptoms of pernicious anaemia are usually insidious in nature and worsen over time. The symptoms and signs are similar to those for other anaemias but may also include neurological symptoms as a result of the vitamin B_{12} deficiency. Some symptoms of anaemia include:

- Fatigue.
- Shortness of breath.
- Dizziness.
- Syncope.
- Angina on effort.
- Palpitations.
- Conjunctival pallor.

Investigations

- Blood tests: FBC, U&Es, LFTs, Coag, iron studies, vitamin B_{12}, Schilling test.

Treatment

- Conservative: patient education.
- Medical: lifelong parenteral vitamin B_{12} replacement.

Complications

- Associated with severe anaemia: tachycardia, palpitations, heart failure.
- Neurological complications: paraesthesia, ataxia, peripheral neuropathy, visual disturbances.
- Stomach cancer.
- Neural tube defects (in pregnant women).
- Infertility (temporary).

MAP 7.4 **Pernicious Anaemia**

Map 7.4 Pernicious Anaemia

What is sickle cell anaemia?

This is an inherited haematological disorder in which red blood cells are sickle in shape. There is increased prevalence in sub-Saharan Africa where there is a high incidence of malaria. The sickle cell shape is thought to confer some protection against *P. falciparum*.

Cause

Autosomal recessive disease (Figure 7.3).

Typically, haemoglobin is made up of four subunits or chains. Each has a protein part, i.e. the globin, and a non-protein part, i.e. the haem (which in turn is made up of iron and protoporphyrin). Adult haemoglobin (HbA) is made from two alpha chains and two beta chains. Each chain contains haem which carries one oxygen molecule loosely and reversibly.

In sickle cell disease there is a defect in the beta-globin chain. This is because of a missense, non-conservative, point mutation where glutamine (hydrophilic) is replaced by valine (hydrophobic) at position 6 on the surface of the beta-globin chain (chromosome 11). The result is HbS and a red blood cell that will change its shape to a sickle shape in a deoxygenated environment. Sickle shaped red blood cells are more likely to have membrane damage and subsequent haemolysis.

MAP 7.5 **Sickle Cell Anaemia**

Investigations

- Prenatal: DNA-based PCR or allele-specific hybridisation (CVS or amniocentesis).
- Postnatal: FBC (decreased RBC count, Hb and Hct), sickle cell screen – sodium metabisulphite test (this decreases the oxygen tension and forces the cell to sickle).
- Peripheral blood smear: sickle cells.
- Gel electrophoresis: HbS.

Treatment

- There is no cure.
- Conservative: patient education, genetic testing, vaccination (flu, *Pneumococcus* and against encapsulated organisms because of functional asplenia), fundus examination for retinopathy.
- Medical: daily folic acid to combat the haemolysis and rapid turnover of cells.
  - For vaso-occlusive disease: follow your local hospital protocol but generally management consists of rehydration, antibiotics, analgesia, hydroxyurea (shifts oxygen dissociation curve to the left, therefore anti-sickling), transfusion.

Complications

- Vaso-occlusive crisis (and symptoms related to any of the organs involved).
- Splenic sequestration.
- Pulmonary hypertension.
- Osteomyelitis (*Salmonella*).
- Avascular necrosis (of femoral head).
- Renal papillary necrosis.
- Acute chest syndrome.
- Blindness.
- Leg ulcers.
- Gallstones (haemolysis).
- Priapism.
- Infection from encapsulated organisms.

FIGURE 7.3 Inheritance Pattern of Sickle Cell Anaemia

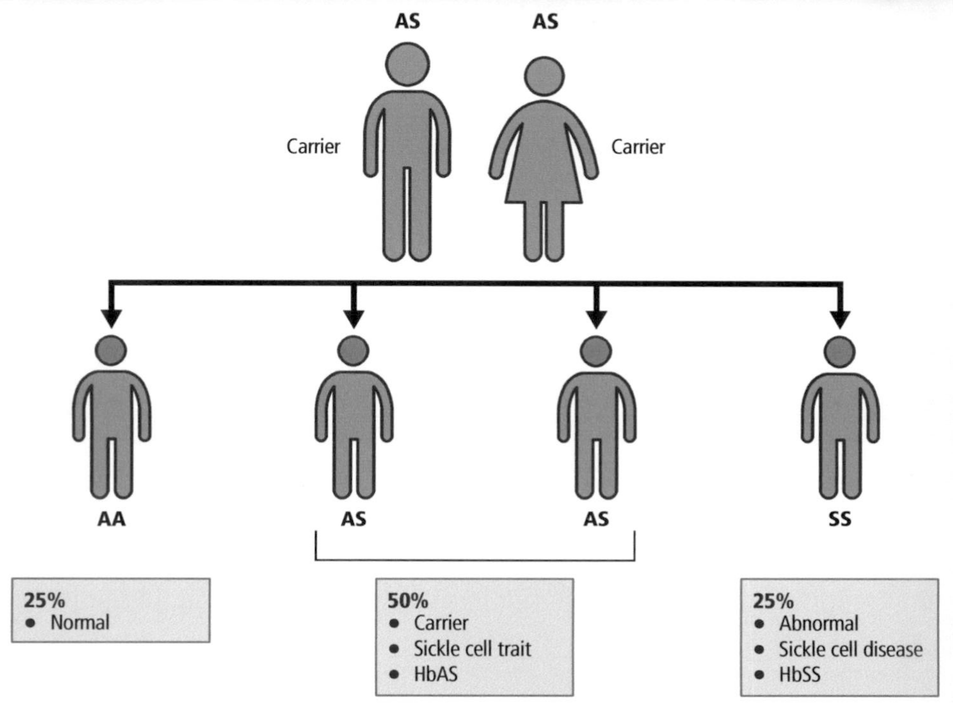

Carrier
AS

AS
Carrier

AA

AS

AS

SS

25%
- Normal

50%
- Carrier
- Sickle cell trait
- HbAS

25%
- Abnormal
- Sickle cell disease
- HbSS

Signs and symptoms

- Symptoms of anaemia: fatigue, malaise, shortness of breath, anaemia on exertion, palpitation.
- Conjunctival pallor.
- Jaundice.
- Hepatosplenomegaly.
- Extramedullary haematopoiesis.
- Symptoms related to vaso-occlusive crisis – this depends on which organ is affected.
  Some examples include:
  ○ Dactylitis.
  ○ Pulmonary hypertension.
  ○ Osteomyelitis (*Salmonella*, because of autosplenectomy there is greater risk from encapsulated organisms).
  ○ Renal papillary necrosis.
  ○ Autosplenectomy.
  ○ Aplastic crisis (parvovirus B19).
  ○ Proliferative retinopathy.
  ○ Stroke.

MAP 7.6 **Thalassaemia**

Map 7.6 Thalassaemia

What is thalassaemia?

Thalassaemias are genetic conditions, inherited in an autosomal recessive pattern, that produce a picture of microcytic anaemia due to a problem in globin chain production. This subsequently alters haemoglobin (Hb) synthesis. Thalassaemia may be classified into α-thalassaemia and β-thalassaemia.

Table 7.2 **Thalassaemia**

Types of thalassaemia	Populations affected	Causes	Investigations	Treatment	Complications
α-thalassaemia	More prominent in African and Asian populations	↓ α-globin synthesis due to α-globin gene mutation on chromosome 16; this subsequently results in excess β-globin production In α-thalassaemia any number between 1 and 4 genes may be deleted: • 1 gene deleted = no significant anaemia • 2 genes deleted = trait disease • 3 genes deleted = HbH disease • 4 genes deleted = death – Bart's hydrops fetalis	Blood films: in α-thalassaemia target cells (or Mexican hat cells) may be seen FBC: • Microcytic, hypochromic anaemia • ↓ MCV • ↓ MCH • Ferritin normal • Iron normal Hb electrophoresis: ↑ HbA$_2$ and ↑ HbF High performance liquid chromatography Radiology: X-ray for bone abnormalities, e.g. frontal bossing	Conservative: patient education, genetic counselling Medical: • Management of α-thalassaemia and β-thalassaemia is based on patient symptoms and overall state of health • Transfusions are usually required when Hb <7 g/dL or when the patient is highly symptomatic	Iron overload Splenomegaly Increased risk of infection Heart failure Arrhythmias Bone abnormalities, e.g. cranial bossing Gallstones

| β-thalassaemia | More prominent in European populations | Point mutation in β-globin chain on chromosome 11; this subsequently results in excess α-globin production

β-thalassaemia may be subdivided into 3 different traits:
1 Minor: usually asymptomatic; carrier state; mild anaemia
2 Intermediate: moderate anaemia; no blood transfusions required
3 Major: aka Cooley's anaemia; abnormalities in all β-globin chains result in severe anaemia; characteristic cranial bossing seen due to extramedullary haematopoiesis | | • Patients who have repeated blood transfusions are at risk of haemo-chromatosis and, therefore, require iron chelation therapy, e.g. desferroxamine

Surgical:
• Splenectomy
• Stem cell transplant |

Table 7.2 Thalassaemia

Figure 7.4 The Coagulation Cascade

FIGURE 7.4 **The Coagulation Cascade**

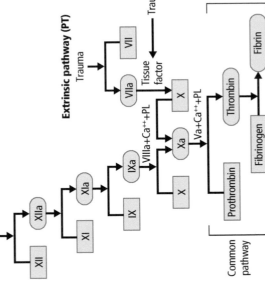

Intrinsic pathway (APTT)

Damaged surface

Kallikrein
Collagen
High molecular weight kininogen (HMWK)

Extrinsic pathway (PT)

Trauma

Trauma

Tissue factor

Common pathway

Key points about factors within the coagulation cascade:

- Factor VII has the shortest half-life.
- Factors V and VIII are the most labile factors. Their activity is lost in stored blood but not in FFP.
- Factor VIII is the only factor that is not synthesised by the liver. It is made by endothelium.
- Factors II, VII, IX and X are vitamin K dependent (along with proteins C and S).
- Factor X is the common point of both pathways.
- Factor XIII helps to cross-link fibrin.

Thrombin is the key to coagulation. It converts fibrinogen to fibrin, it activates factors V and VIII and it stimulates platelets. Fibrin links platelets together. Binding of GPIIb/IIIa promotes platelet plug formation.

Coagulation measurements:

PT measures factors II, V, VII, X and fibrinogen. It is the best marker of synthetic liver function.
PTT measures most factors except VII and XIII.

Problem	PT	APTT
Platelet problem	Normal	Normal
Factor VII problem	Increased	Normal
Common pathway problem	Increased	Increased
Intrinsic pathway problem	Normal	Increased
Extrinsic pathway problem	Increased	Normal

Figure 7.4 The Coagulation Cascade

Map 7.7 Bleeding Disorders

HAEMOPHILIA

What is haemophilia?

This is an inherited condition that impairs the body's ability to coagulate the blood.

Causes

This is a hereditary condition. There are two forms of haemophilia:

- Type A: lack of factor VIII.
- Type B: lack of factor IX.

Investigations

- Normal prothrombin time, ↑ partial thromboplastin time.

Treatment

- Conservative: patient education. Avoid aspirin, NSAIDs, heparin and warfarin.
- Medical: replace deficient clotting factor with regular infusions.

CLOT FORMATION

This consists of 4 steps. Defects in steps 2–4 may lead to a bleeding disorder.

1. Vessel constriction.
2. Platelet adhesion and aggregation: Glanzmann's thrombasthenia, von Willebrand's disease, Bernard–Soulier syndrome.
3. Blood coagulation: haemophilia.
4. Fibrinolysis: antiplasmin deficiency.

BERNARD–SOULIER SYNDROME

What is Bernard–Soulier syndrome?

This is an autosomal recessive bleeding disorder.

Causes

This is a hereditary condition that leads to deficiency of glycoprotein (Gp) Ib.

Investigations

- ↑ Bleeding time, normal or ↓ platelet count.

Treatment

- Conservative: patient education.
- Medical:
  - Desmopressin may decrease bleeding time.
  - Recombinant activated factor VII.

MAP 7.7 Bleeding Disorders

VITAMIN K INSUFFICIENCY

What is vitamin K insuffiency?

This avitaminosis occurs when there is decreased vitamin K_1 or vitamin K_2 or both. This results in:

- ↓ Synthesis of factors II, VII, IX and X.
- ↓ Synthesis of proteins C and S.

Causes

- Drugs, e.g. warfarin.
- Malnutrition.
- Malabsorption.
- Alcoholism.
- Cystic fibrosis.
- Chronic kidney injury.
- Cholestatic disease.

Investigations

- ↑ Prothrombin time, normal or ↑ partial thromboplastin time.

Treatment

- Conservative – patient education. Dietary advice about food rich in vitamin K
- Medical – treat cause. Vitamin K supplements.

GLANZMANN'S THROMBASTHENIA

What is Glanzmann's thrombasthenia?

This is a rare autosomal recessive or acquired autoimmune condition in which platelets are deficient in GpIIb/IIIa. GpIIb/IIIa binds fibrinogen.

Causes

Disease of hereditary or acquired autoimmune cause.

Investigations

- ↑ Bleeding time.

Treatment

- Conservative: patient education. Avoid aspirin and nonsteroidal anti-inflammatory drugs (NSAIDs).
- Medical:
  ○ Desmopressin.
  ○ Recombinant activated factor VII.

VON WILLEBRAND'S DISEASE

What is von Willebrand's disease?

This is the most common hereditary coagulation disorder, which involves a defect in von Willebrand's factor (VWF). The function of VWF is to bind Gplb receptor on platelets to subendothelial collagen.

Causes

Hereditary condition. There are many different types of von Willebrand's disease, but the most common are type 1, type 2, type 3 and type Normandy.

Investigations

- ↑ Activated partial thromboplastin time,
- ↑ Bleeding time, normal prothrombin time, ↓ VWF antigen, ↓ factor VIIIc.

Treatment

- Conservative: patient education. Avoid aspirin and NSAIDs.
- Medical: desmopressin may be useful, but is not helpful in type 3 von Willebrand's disease.

Map 7.8 Leukaemia

What is leukaemia?

Leukaemias describe malignancies arising from bone marrow stem cells. They are classified into lymphoid and myeloid neoplasms, which may present chronically or acutely.

The 4 classifications are:

1 Acute lymphoblastic leukaemia (ALL).
2 Chronic lymphocytic leukaemia (CLL).
3 Acute myeloid leukaemia (AML).
4 Chronic myeloid leukaemia (CML).

The malignant cells replace most of the normal bone marrow cells before entering the peripheral blood and they metastasise.

Leukaemias are more common in males than females and are more common in adults than children.

ALL is the commonest leukaemia and the most common cancer in children. Sometimes, the type of leukaemia may be predicted based on the age of the patient:
Newborn–14 years: ALL.
40–60 years: AML or CML.
>60 years: CLL.

Causes

Neoplasm	Cause	Comment
ALL	Possibly a genetic susceptibility coupled with an environmental trigger	Commonest cancer in children Often spreads to central nervous system Associations – **DIP**: ● **D**own's syndrome ● **I**onising radiation ● **P**regnancy
CLL	Exact cause unknown	Usually affects adults over 60 years old Affects B lymphocytes Positive ZAP-70 marker is associated with a worse prognosis
AML	Exact cause unknown Risk factors include: ● Myeloproliferative disease ● Alkylating agents ● Ionising radiation exposure ● Down's syndrome	Commonest leukaemia in adults Rapidly progressing Auer rods on microscopy are diagnostic
CML	Exact cause unknown Risk factor: ionising radiation exposure	Usually affects males 40–60 years old 80% associated with the Philadelphia chromosome t[9;22], forming *BCR-ABL* fusion gene

MAP 7.8 **Leukaemia**

Signs and symptoms

Neoplasm	Clinical features
ALL	Bone marrow failure Bruising Shortness of breath Purpura Malaise Weight loss Night sweats
CLL	Asymptomatic Bone marrow failure Non-tender lymphadenopathy Hepatosplenomegaly Malaise Weight loss Night sweats
AML	Bone marrow failure Malaise Weight loss Night sweats
CML	Bone marrow failure Hepatosplenomegaly Malaise Weight loss Night sweats

Investigations

- Bloods: FBC, WCC, platelets, U&Es, LFTs, ESR, CRP.
- Bone marrow biopsy, lymph node biopsy.
- Radiology: X-ray, ultrasound scan, CT scan, MRI.
- AML and ALL are classified using the French–American–British (FAB) classification.

Complications

- Death.
- Increased risk of infection.
- Haemorrhage: pulmonary, intracranial.
- Depression.
- Complication of chemotherapy.

Treatment

Treatment	ALL	CLL	AML	CML
Conservative	Patient education; refer to Macmillan nurses			
Medical	Induce remission and maintenance To induce remission: • Dexamethasone • Vincristine • Anthracycline antibiotics • Cyclophosphamide Maintenance: • Methotrexate • Mercaptopurine • Cytarabine • Hydrocortisone	Chlorambucil Fludarabine Rituximab Prednisolone Cyclophosphamide	Patients <60 years: chemotherapy with an anthracycline and cytarabine or methotrexate Patients >60 years: palliative anthracycline, cytarabine or mitoxantrone If M3-type AML, i.e. acute promyelocytic leukaemia (APML), then add all-trans retinoic acid to the therapeutic regimen	Imatinib Patients <60 years may be considered for allogeneic stem cell transplantation Other treatments include: interferon-alpha, vincristine, prednisolone, cytarabine and daunorubicin

Map 7.8 Leukaemia

What are acute lymphoblastic leukaemia (ALL) and acute myeloid leukaemia (AML)?

Acute leukaemia is when there are >20% blasts in the bone marrow. It is a monoclonal disorder of the early haematopoietic stem cells, i.e. early lymphoid (ALL) or early myeloid (AML) lines. These cells lose their ability to differentiate but they replicate abnormally. Therefore, the proliferating blasts end up replacing most of the bone marrow cells meaning that patients are prone to infections (decreased WCC), fatigue/anaemia (decreased RBC count) and bleeding (decreased platelets).

Signs and symptoms

- Symptoms of anaemia: fatigue, malaise, shortness of breath, anaemia on exertion, palpitation.
- Recurrent infection.
- Bruising easily/mucosal bleeding.
- Lymphadenopathy.
- Hepatosplenomegaly.
- Symptoms of raised intracranial pressure, e.g. headache, cranial nerve palsies, papilloedema.
- Testicular enlargement.

Causes

The exact cause of ALL and AML is unknown. They are thought to be associated with genetic and environmental risk factors. AML tends to affect patients aged in the 40s, whereas ALL tends to affect young adults and children.
The risk factors are detailed below.

Risk factors for ALL and AML

- Antineoplastic agents.
- Ionising radiation.
- Benzene exposure.
- Multiple myeloma.
- Hodgkin's lymphoma.
- ALL has increased association with Down's syndrome and Fanconi anaemia.
- AML has increased association with Down's syndrome, Turner's syndrome and Klinefelter's syndrome.

MAP 7.9 **The Acute Leukaemias** Acute lymphoblastic Leukaemia (ALL) and Acute Myeloid Leukaemia (AML)

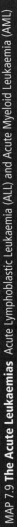

Investigations

- Bloods: FBC, U&Es, LFTs, Coag, iron studies.
- Cytogenic studies (karyotype).
- Cell surface markers – cluster of differentiation (CD), flow cytometry and immunophenotyping.
- Cytochemical analysis – periodic acid stain (PAS), peroxidase, esterase, Sudan Black stain.
- Auer rods are associated with AML (myeloperoxidase positive).
- ALL is positive for terminal deoxynucleotidyltransferase (TdT). This is a DNA polymerase.

- Morphological analysis: peripheral blood smear, % blasts.
- Molecular markers.

Investigation	ALL	AML
Peripheral blood smear	Lymphoblasts – medium sized, agranular, scanty cytoplasm, increase nuclear:cytoplasmic ratio	Myeloid blasts: • Myeloblasts – Auer rods, more granules myeloperoxidase positive • Monoblasts – fewer granules, no Auer rods
Bone marrow biopsy	Hypercellular, blasts >20%	Hypercellular, blasts >20%
Morphological analysis	Lymphoblasts	Myeloid blasts
Cytogenic studies (karyotype)	t[9;22] and t[12;21]	t[8;21] (commonest) and t[15;17] = good prognosis inv(16) = good prognosis t[19;11] = intermediate prognosis inv(3), monosomy 7 and 5q deletion = poor prognosis
Cell surface markers	B cell: CD10, 19 and 20 T cell: CD3, 4, 5, 6, 7, 8	CD34, CD38, CD123, TIM3, CD25, CD32 and CD96
Cell surface markers	PAS positive TdT positive Esterase negative	TdT negative Myeloperoxidase positive

Continued overleaf

Map 7.9 The Acute Leukaemias

Classifications

- ALL is classified into:
  - Pre-B ALL – commonest.
    - More common in children.
    - Associated with Down's syndrome.
    - CD10 positive, CD19 positive, CD20 positive.
    - Translocations: t[9;22] = bad prognosis, t[12;21] = good prognosis.
  - B cell ALL.
    - Translocations: t[8;14] = Burkitt's leukaemia, t[8;22], t[2;8].
  - T cell ALL.
    - Usually in young adults.
    - Associated with a mediastinal mass.
    - CD3 positive, CD7 positive.
- AML has a French–American–British subclassification:
  - M0: undifferentiated myeloblasts.
  - M1: myelocytic leukaemia without differentiation.
  - M2: myelocytic leukaemia with differentiation.
  - M3: acute promyelocytic leukaemia.
    - t[15;17] promyelocytic leukaemia gene and retinoic acid receptor alpha gene.
    - Associated with DIC.
    - Has a very good prognosis and can treat with all-trans retinoic acid (ATRA).
  - M4: acute myelocytic leukaemia.
  - M5: acute monocytic leukaemia proliferation of monoblasts.
  - M6: acute erythroblastic leukaemia (myeloblasts and proerythroblasts).
  - M7: acute megakaryocytic leukaemia (myeloblasts and megakaryocytes).

Complications

- Tumour lysis syndrome: hyperkalaemia, increased uric acid (AKI), hyperphosphataemia.
- High cell turnover: folate deficiency (megaloblastic anaemia), hyperkalaemia (arrythmias), increased uric acid (AKI), hyperphosphataemia.
- Neurocognitive dysfunction.
- Complications of chemotherapy.
- Death.

Poor prognostic indicators for ALL

- Age >60 years.
- WCC >100,000.
- Mature B cell or early T cell classification.
- Philadelphia chromosome t[9;22].
- *MLL-AF4* fusion gene t[4;11].

Poor prognostic indicators for AML

- Age >60 years.
- WCC >100,000.
- Secondary AML, i.e. had another disease of the bone marrow which transformed into AML, e.g. MDS.
- *FLT3* mutation.

MAP 7.9 **The Acute Leukaemias** (*Continued*)

Treatment for ALL

- Conservative: patient education, cancer support nurses, sperm banking.
- Medical:
  - Induction: this aims to induce remission and suppresses all cell lines. The aim is to reduce blasts to an undetectable level; however, there are two main problems encountered: 1. resistance and 2. infection risk. Example agents include prednisolone and vincristine, anthracycline antibiotics, L-asparaginase. The exact regimen needs to be discussed at MDT with haematology/oncology.
    - Myeloid growth factor – may reduce the time spent in the neutropenic state and helps to reduce morbidity as well as hospital stay; however, it does not reduce mortality.
    - Patients may receive blood and platelet transfusions.
    - If neutropenic sepsis occurs, then follow local guidelines and perform Sepsis Six.

    Patients are at risk of tumour lysis syndrome: give good hydration and allopurinol.
  - Consolidation (followed by maintenance): aims to prolong remission and increase survival. Example agents include methotrexate, cyclophosphamide, cytarabine. The exact regimen needs to be discussed at MDT with haematology/oncology. If t[9;22] in ALL, then can try tyrosine kinase inhibitor imatinib.
    - Bone marrow transplant is considered in younger individuals.
    - CNS prophylaxis and testicles: CNS – intrathecal methotrexate +/– cranial radiation; testes – radiation.

Treatment for AML

- Conservative: patient education, cancer support nurses, sperm banking.
- Medical:
  - Induction; this aims to induce remission and suppresses all cell lines. The aim is to reduce blasts to an undetectable level; however, there are two main problems encountered: 1. resistance and 2. infection risk. Example agents include cytosine arabinoside and an anthracycline antibiotic. The exact regimen needs to be discussed at MDT with haematology/oncology.
    - Myeloid growth factor – may reduce the time spent in the neutropenic state and helps to reduce morbidity as well as hospital stay; however, it does not reduce mortality.
    - Patients may receive blood and platelet transfusions.
    - If neutropenic sepsis occurs, then follow local guidelines and perform Sepsis Six.
    - Patients are at risk of tumour lysis syndrome: give good hydration and allopurinol.
  - Consolidation (followed by maintenance); aims to prolong remission and increase survival. Example agents include cytosine arabinoside and an anthracycline antibiotic.

    The exact regimen needs to be discussed at MDT with haematology/ oncology.
    - Allogenic stem cell transplants in individuals aged <60 years.
    - If AML M3: acute promyelocytic leukaemia then consider treatment with ATRA.

Map 7.9 The Acute Leukaemias

Map 7.10 The Chronic Leukaemias

MAP 7.10 **The Chronic Leukaemias** Chronic Lymphocytic Leukaemia (CLL) and Chronic Myelogenous Leukaemia (CML)

What are chronic lymphocytic leukaemia (CLL) and chronic myelogenous leukaemia (CML)?

Chronic leukaemias are monoclonal disorders of small, mature haematopoietic stem cells. These cells are dysfunctional. Onset tends to be insidious in older patients. There are <10% blasts.

CML is a malignancy of the bone marrow stem cells where there is proliferation of all white blood cells except for the lymphocytes as it is from the myeloid lineage (especially neutrophils). It is associated with the translocation t(9;22), i.e. the Philadelphia chromosome, forming *BCR-ABL* fusion gene. Note that this chromosome can be present in some patients with ALL.

CLL is a lymphoproliferative disorder in which cells are morphologically mature but they are dysfunctional. Typically asymptomatic and affects those >60 years old. Affects males more than females.

Signs and symptoms
- Constitutional features: weight loss, sweating, fevers.
- Generalised lymphadenopathy.
- Abdominal pain.
- Hepatosplenomegaly.
- Symptoms associated with bone marrow failure, e.g. anaemia, infection, bleeding.

Phases of CML
- Chronic phase: asymptomatic or mild symptoms. Responds well to imatinib.
- Accelerated phase: splenomegaly, basophilia.
- Blast crisis: transformation into an acute leukaemia AML in 70%. It is generally refractory to treatment.

Staging of CLL (the Rai system)
0 – lymphocytosis of blood and marrow.
I – lymphocytosis and lymphadenopathy.
II – lymphocytosis with hepatosplenomegaly.
III – stage 0–II with haemoglobin <11 g/dL.
IV – stage 0–III with platelets <100 × 10^9/L.
Please see: https://www.researchgate.net/figure/Chronic-lymphocytic-leukemia-Rai-staging-system_tbl2_15585634

Investigations

- Bloods: FBC, U&Es, LFTs, Coag, iron studies.
- Morphological analysis: peripheral blood smear, % blasts.
- Cytogenic studies (karyotype): FISH or PCR.
- Bone marrow biopsy.
- RNA analysis for BCR-ABL fusion protein.

Investigation	CML	CLL
Peripheral blood smear	Normocytic anaemia or megaloblastic anaemia if folate deficiency Thrombocytosis <10% blasts Leukaemic cells – all stages of development Basophilia – more with progression of disease	Lymphocytosis 'Smudge' cells Thrombocytopenia <10% blasts
Bone marrow biopsy	Hypercellular bone marrow with myeloid hyperplasia <10% blasts	Lymphocytes >30% <10% blasts
Cytogenic studies (karyotype)	t[9;22]	Zeta-chain-associated protein kinase 70 (ZAP 70) positive is associated with a poorer prognosis

Treatment

- Conservative: patient education, cancer support nurse.
- Medical:
  - CML: tyrosine kinase inhibitor imatinib.
  - CLL: focus is on supportive measures rather than a curative approach.
    If early stage then no treatment as no increased survival benefit. Apply a watchful waiting approach.
  - If symptomatic or evidence of bone marrow failure, then consider chemotherapy. Example regimens include FCR – fludarabine, cyclophosphamide and rituximab – but this would need to be discussed with haematology/oncology at MDT.
  - If lymphadenopathy then debulking radiotherapy may be considered.
    Stem cell transplant is a last resort.

Complications

- Frequent infections.
- Transformation into an acute leukaemia.
- Side effects of chemotherapy.
- Side effects of bone marrow failure; bleeding, infection, anaemia.
- Death.

Map 7.10 The Chronic Leukaemias

Map 7.11 Hodgkin's vs. Non-Hodgkin's Lymphoma

MAP 7.11
Hodgkin's vs. Non-Hodgkin's Lymphoma

HODGKIN'S LYMPHOMA
What is Hodgkin's lymphoma?
This is a group of uncommon malignancies; the 4 most common histological subtypes are:

1 Lymphocyte-predominant.
2 Nodular sclerosing.
3 Mixed cellularity.
4 Lymphocyte-depleted.

Cause
Exact cause is unknown.
Risk factors include:

- Male sex.
- Infection with Epstein–Barr virus (EBV).
- Immunosuppression, e.g. HIV patients.
- Exotoxin exposure.

Signs and symptoms
- Painless lymphadenopathy.
- Unintentional weight loss.
- Fever (constitutional 'B signs': fever >38°C, night sweats, weight loss).

NON-HODGKIN'S LYMPHOMA
What is non-Hodgkin's lymphoma?
This is a group of malignancies that are either B cell or T cell in origin.

B cell neoplasms	T cell neoplasms
Burkitt's lymphoma:	Adult T cell lymphoma; caused by human
• Associated with EBV	T-lymphotrophic virus-1 (HTLV-1)
• t[8;14]	Sézary's syndrome
Diffuse large B cell lymphoma	
Mantle cell lymphoma: t[11;14]	
Follicular lymphoma:	
• t[14;18]	
• *BCL-2* expression	

Cause
Exact cause is unknown.
Risk factors include:

- Male sex.
- Infection, e.g. EBV, *Helicobacter pylori*, human herpes virus (HHV)-8, hepatitis C.
- Immunosuppression, e.g. HIV patients.

- Dyspnoea.
- Splenomegaly.
- Hepatomegaly.

Investigations
- Bloods: FBC, WCC, U&Es, CRP, ESR, lactate dehydrogenase, creatinine, alkaline phosphatase, serum cytokine levels.
- Histology: Reed–Sternberg cells are seen.
- Radiology: X-ray, CT scan, PET scan.
- Other: lymph node biopsy (Ann Arbor classification).

Treatment
- Conservative: patient education and referral to Macmillan nurses.
- Medical: depends on Ann Arbor classification; AVBD regimen: doxorubicin, vinblastine, bleomycin, dacarbazine; BEACOPP regimen: bleomycin, etoposide, doxorubicin, cyclophosphamide, vincristine, procarbazine, prednisolone.

Complications
- Increased risk of infection.
- Recurrence and metastasis.
- Increased risk of cardiovascular disease.
- Complications of chemotherapy.
- Neurological complications.

Signs and symptoms
- Painless lymphadenopathy.
- Unintentional weight loss.
- Fever.
- Dyspnoea.
- Splenomegaly.
- Hepatomegaly.

Investigations
- Bloods: FBC, WCC, U&Es, CRP, ESR, lactate dehydrogenase, creatinine, alkaline phosphatase, serum cytokine levels, soluble CD25 level.
- Radiology: X-ray, CT scan, PET scan.
- Other: lymph node biopsy (Ann Arbor classification).

Treatment
- Conservative: patient education and referral to Macmillan nurses.
- Medical: depends on causes and severity (Ann Arbor classification); R-CHOP regimen: rituximab, cyclophosphamide, hydroxydaunomycin, vincristine, prednisolone; other agents used are cisplatin, etoposide and methotrexate.

Complications
- Increased risk of infection.
- Recurrence and metastasis.
- Increased risk of cardiovascular disease.
- Complications of chemotherapy.
- Neurological complications.

Map 7.11 Hodgkin's vs. Non-Hodgkin's Lymphoma

Map 7.12 Myeloma

What is myeloma?

This is a malignant neoplasm of the plasma cells.

Causes

Exact cause is unknown.
Risk factors include:

- Monoclonal gammopathy of unknown significance.
- Pernicious anaemia.
- History of thyroid cancer.
- Exposure to certain exotoxins, e.g. benzene, Agent Orange.
- Past history of radiation exposure.

Signs and symptoms

- Fatigue.
- Unintentional weight loss.
- Pathological fractures.
- Vertebral collapse (may lead to spinal cord compression).
- Hypercalcaemia.
- Anaemia.
- Infection.
- Renal impairment.
- Bruising.

Investigations

- Bloods: FBC (normocytic, normochromic anaemia), U&Es, creatinine, LFTs, ESR, CRP, calcium levels, alkaline phosphatase, beta$_2$ microglobulin.
- Blood film: rouleaux formation.
- Serum and urine electrophoresis: paraprotein (M protein), Bence Jones proteinuria.
- Bone marrow biopsy.
- Radiology:
  ○ X-ray for bone deformities, e.g. pepper-pot skull and generalised skeletal osteopaenia.
  ○ MRI scan may be useful.

Complications

- Spinal cord compression.
- Pathological fracture.
- Hypercalcaemia.
- Acute kidney injury.
- Increased risk of infection.
- Anaemia.

MAP 7.12 **Myeloma**

Treatment

- Conservative: patient education. Refer to Macmillan nurses.
- Medical: medical therapy in multiple myeloma depends on the age of the patient and their state of health. If they are <70 years and without significant comorbidities then they are eligible for autologous bone marrow transplant, which is the most effective treatment. This involves an induction phase using the VAD regimen: vincristine, doxorubicin, dexamethasone. After transplant the patient receives long-term therapy with melphalan.
  ○ Patients who are ineligible for autologous bone marrow transplant receive long-term treatment with melphalan and prednisolone.
  ○ Other medical therapy is targeted to treating symptoms: analgesia, bisphosphonates, prednisolone, blood transfusion.
  ○ Radiotherapy may be required to treat bone pain and spinal cord compression.
- Surgical: kyphoplasty may be required.

Map 8.1   Arthritis

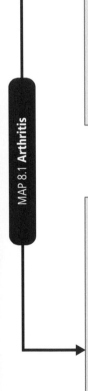

MAP 8.1 **Arthritis**

RHEUMATOID ARTHRITIS (RA)

What is RA?

This is a chronic, autoimmune, type III hypersensitivity reaction that principally affects the joints but may also affect other organs. Joint involvement is characterised by symmetrical deformation with pain that is worse in the morning.

Cause

The exact cause of RA is unknown, but it is thought to involve a type III hypersensitivity reaction. This condition is associated with HLA-DR4 and HLA-DR1.

Signs and symptoms

- Hands: Z deformity, boutonnière deformity, swan neck deformity, ulnar deviation, subluxation of the fingers, Raynaud's phenomenon.
- Wrist: carpal tunnel syndrome.
- Feet: subluxation of the toes, hammer toe deformity.
- Skin: rheumatoid nodule, vasculitis.
- Cardiovascular: atherosclerosis is increased in RA.
- Respiratory: pulmonary fibrosis.
- Bones: osteoporosis.
- Pain and stiffness.

OSTEOARTHRITIS (OA)

What is OA?

This is a degenerative arthritis affecting synovial joints and is characterised by cartilage degeneration, the associated response of the periarticular tissue and pain that is typically worse at the end of the day.

Causes

Damage to the joints and general wear and tear of the joint over time are thought to be the primary cause of OA. There are certain factors that increase the risk of OA such as:

- Increased age.
- Obesity.
- Trauma to the joint.
- Conditions such as haemochromatosis and Ehlers–Danlos syndrome.

Signs and symptoms

- Pain and stiffness.
- Swelling around the joints involved.
- Crepitus.
- Heberden's nodes at distal interphalangeal (DIP) joints. Remember they are the 'outer Hebrides'.
- Bouchard's nodes at proximal interphalangeal (PIP) joints.

Investigations

- Bloods:
  - 80% test positive for rheumatoid factor.
  - ESR and CRP raised.
  - Cyclic citrullinated peptide (CCP) antibodies. If positive this is suggestive of erosive disease.
- Radiology: radiological signs of RA are visualised on plain film:
  - Bony erosion.
  - Subluxation.
  - Carpal instability.
  - Joint involvement of metacarpophalangeal joint (MCPJ) and metatarsophalangeal joint (MTPJ).
  - Periarticular osteoporosis.

Treatment

- Conservative: patient education. Encourage exercise. Refer to physiotherapy and assess activities of daily living (ADLs).
- Medical: glucocorticoids, disease-modifying antirheumatic drugs (DMARDs), e.g. gold salts, methotrexate, sulfasalazine. Anticytokine therapies may be considered in patients intolerant of methotrexate.
- Surgery: excision arthroplasty or replacement may be considered in severely affected joints.

Complications

- Carpal tunnel syndrome.
- Pericarditis.
- Cervical myopathy.
- Tendon rupture.
- Sjögren's syndrome.

Investigations

- Bloods: usually are not diagnostic but may be relevant when OA is related to another condition such as haemochromatosis.
- Radiology: radiological signs: **LOSS**
  - **L**oss of joint space.
  - **O**steophytes.
  - **S**ubchondral cysts.
  - **S**clerosis.

Treatment

- Conservative: patient education. Encourage exercise and weight loss.
- Medical:
  - Analgesia, e.g. paracetamol or nonsteroidal anti-inflammatory drugs.
  - Gels such as capsaicin may be useful.
  - Steroid injections.
- Surgical: arthroplasty.

Complications

- Increased risk of gout.
- Chondrocalcinosis.

Map 8.2 Spondyloarthropathies

REACTIVE ARTHRITIS

What is reactive arthritis?

This is an asymmetrical arthritis that occurs post-gastrointestinal or urogenital infection.

Causes

The exact cause and pathophysiology of this condition is not known.

However, it often occurs after an infection, typically a sexually transmitted infection or an infection of the gastrointestinal tract.

Signs and symptoms

- Urethritis.
- Arthritis: pain and stiffness.
- Uveitis/conjunctivitis.

Investigations

- Bloods: seronegative for rheumatoid factor. Blood cultures. Look for infectious cause.
- Radiology: X-ray of affected joint (assesses severity).

Treatment

- Conservative: patient education. Refer to physiotherapy.
- Medical: analgesia nonsteroidal anti-inflammatory drugs (NSAIDs) and disease-modifying antirheumatic drugs (DMARDs), e.g. sulfasalazine (first line).

Complications

- Arrhythmia.
- Uveitis.
- Aortic insufficiency.

Remember PEAR:

- **P**soriatic arthritis.
- **E**nteropathic arthropathies.
- **A**nkylosing spondylitis.
- **R**eactive arthritis.

MAP 8.2 **Spondyloarthropathies**

PSORIATIC ARTHRITIS

What is psoriatic arthritis?

This is an inflammatory arthritis that is associated with the skin condition psoriasis. It is associated with HLA-B27. The signs and symptoms also depend on how and where the joints are affected. Accordingly, psoriatic arthritis may be split into 5 subtypes:

1. Asymmetrical oligoarthritis (distal and proximal interphalangeal joints).
2. Symmetrical rheumatoid-like arthropathy.
3. Ankylosing spondylitis variant.
4. Polyarteritis with skin and nail changes.
5. Arthritis mutilans.

Causes

The exact cause is unknown. It is thought to be due to an inflammatory process coupled with genetic involvement of the *HLA-B27* gene.
The greatest risk factor is a family history of psoriasis.

Signs and symptoms

- Psoriasis: well-demarcated salmon-pink plaques with evidence of scaling. These plaques are usually present on the extensor surfaces (chronic plaque psoriasis) but sometimes smaller plaques may occur in a raindrop pattern over the torso. This is called guttate psoriasis and is often preceded by an upper respiratory tract infection/sore throat that is caused by *Streptococcus*.
- Joint pain and stiffness.
- Swelling of affected joints.
- Nail changes: there are 4 nail changes noted in psoriasis: yellowing of the nail, onycholysis, pitting and subungual hyperkeratosis.

Continued overleaf

ENTEROPATHIC ARTHROPATHIES

What are enteropathic arthropathies?

This is an arthritis that develops in association with inflammatory bowel disease (IBD). It is indistinguishable from reactive arthritis.

Causes

The exact cause and pathophysiology of this condition are not known. However, it is thought to be associated with HLA-B27.

Signs and symptoms

- Those of IBD, see page 46.
- Spondylitis.
- Sacroiliitis.
- Peripheral arthritis: usually of large joints.

Investigations

- Those for IBD, see page 46.
- Radiology: X-ray of affected joint. Assess severity.

Treatment

- Analgesia (NSAIDs).
- Treatment of IBD, see page 46.

Complications

- Severely decreased mobility with axial involvement.

Map 8.2 Spondyloarthropathies

Map 8.2 Spondyloarthropathies

ANKYLOSING SPONDYLITIS

What is ankylosing spondylitis?

This is a chronic inflammatory disease of the spine and sacroiliac joints. There is predominance in young males and the condition is associated with HLA-B27 (positive in 95%).

Causes

The exact cause and pathophysiology of this condition are not known.
However, it is thought to be associated with HLA-B27.

Signs and symptoms

- Question mark posture.
- Bamboo spine: due to calcification of ligaments.
- Pain and stiffness: symptoms improve with exercise.

Investigations

- Bloods: seronegative for rheumatoid factor.
- Radiology: CXR and MRI assess changes in the spine.

Treatment

- Conservative: patient education. Refer to physiotherapy.
- Medical: analgesia (NSAIDs) and DMARDs, e.g. sulfasalazine (first line).
- Surgical: corrective spinal surgery.

Complications

- Osteoprosis.
- Spinal fractures.
- Increased risk of cardiovascular disease, e.g. stroke and myocardial infarction.

PSORIATIC ARTHRITIS (Continued)

Investigations

- Psoriasis is a clinical diagnosis.
- Bloods: seronegative for rheumatoid factor.
- Radiology: 'pencil-in-cup' deformity on hand X-ray. X-ray of affected joints to assess severity.

Treatment

- Conservative: patient education. Refer to physiotherapy. Explain to patients that psoriasis does not have a cure and control of the disease is more realistic.
- Medical: analgesia (nonsteroidal anti-inflammatory drugs [NSAIDs]) and disease-modifying antirheumatic drugs (DMARDs), e.g. methotrexate (first line). Manage psoriasis.
- Surgery: rarely joint replacement.

Complications

- Neurological manifestations if atlanto-axial joint involvement.
- Joint destruction.

MAP 8.2 **Spondyloarthropathies** (Continued)

What is gout?

Gout is an inflammatory crystal monoarthropathy caused by the deposition of urate crystals as a result of overproduction or underexcretion of uric acid. These monosodium urate crystals often precipitate in the metatarsophalangeal joint (MTPJ). Gout involving the big toe is known as a podagra.

Causes

There are many causes of gout but essentially anything that increases urate levels may be the underlying cause. Some examples include,

Horrific **DELAY**:

- **H**yperuricaemia, **H**ereditary.
- **D**iuretics (thiazides).
- **E**thanol.
- **L**eukaemia.
- ren**A**l impairment.
- associated with Lesch–N**Y**han syndrome.

Hyperuricaemia is defined as a level >7 mg/dL (420 μmol/L).

Signs and symptoms

- Calor, dolor, rubor and tumour (heat, pain, redness and swelling) of the affected joint, which is usually the MTPJ in 50% of patients.
- Tophi (urate deposits) may be present on tendon surfaces, e.g. the elbow, or visible on the ear.
- Patients may have symptoms of renal calculi.

Investigations

- Bloods: serum urate levels, FBC, WCC, U&Es, creatinine, ESR, CRP.
- GFR: assess kidney function.
- Synovial fluid analysis: positively birefringent monosodium urate crystals.

Continued overleaf

Map 8.3 Gout

MAP 8.3 **Gout** (*Continued*)

Complications
- Joint damage.
- Renal calculi.
- Tophi formation.

Treatment
- Conservative: patient education. Lifestyle advice, e.g. encourage alcohol reduction and a low purine diet. Review medications that the patient is taking and stop causative agents, e.g. thiazide diuretics, if possible.
- Medical:
  - Analgesia.
  - Acute: colchicine and steroids.
  - Chronic: allopurinol. Febuxostat may be used if allopurinol is not tolerated by the patient.

When to start allopurinol? Need 2 or more attacks per year to commence treatment. It should not be initiated during an attack as it can worsen symptoms.

Pseudogout vs. gout

Characteristic	Pseudogout	Gout
Joints affected	Larger proximal	Classically 1st MTPJ
Crystal type	Calcium pyrophosphate crystals	Sodium urate crystals
Crystal shape	Rhomboid	Needle
Light microscopy	Negative birefringence	Strongly positive birefringence

MAP 8.4 Metabolic Bone Disease

OSTEOPOROSIS

What is osteoporosis?

This is a bone disease that is characterised by low bone mineral density. This is caused by altered bone microarchitecture and predisposes the patient to fractures. Osteoporosis may be primary (related to aging and decreased sex hormones) or secondary (associated with drug use, e.g. corticosteroids, PPIs, chemotherapy agents).

Causes

This disease is caused by alteration in the bone architecture. There are many risk factors associated with osteoporosis, which one can remember as **OSTEOPOROSIS**:

- l**O**w calcium intake.
- **S**eizure medications.
- **T**hin build.
- **E**thanol.
- hyp**O**gonadism.
- **P**revious fracture.
- thyr**O**id excess.
- **R**ace (increased in white Europeans).
- **O**ther relatives with osteoporosis, **O**ld (age >55 years).
- **S**teroids.
- **I**nactivity.
- **S**moking, **S**ex (female). *Continued overleaf*

OSTEOMALACIA

What is osteomalacia?

This is a metabolic bone disorder characterised by low mineral bone content and deficient vitamin D. This leads to soft bones; however, the amount of bone is normal. In children this condition is called rickets.

Causes

Remember **REVOLT**:

- **RE**sistance to vitamin D.
- **V**itamin D deficiency.
- **O**steodystrophy (renal).
- **L**iver disease.
- **T**umour-induced osteomalacia.

Signs and symptoms

- Bone pain.
- Myalgia.
- Pathological fracture.

Investigations

- Bloods: FBC, U&Es, LFTs, TFTs, glucose, serum calcium, serum phosphate, alkaline phosphatase, PTH and vitamin D levels.
- Radiology: X-ray to assess fractures.

Continued overleaf

Map 8.4 Metabolic Bone Disease

Map 8.4 Metabolic Bone Disease

OSTEOMALACIA (*Continued*)

Treatment
- Conservative: patient education. Dietary advice concerning calcium and vitamin D intake.
- Medical: vitamin D supplements, e.g. cholecalciferol and calcitriol.

Complications
- Increased risk of fracture.

OSTEOPOROSIS (*Continued*)

Signs and symptoms
- Loss of height.
- Dowager's hump (increasing kyphosis).
- Low impact fractures.

Investigations
- Bloods: calcium, phosphate, ALP, TFTs, vitamin D levels.
- Bone density DEXA scan.
- X-ray investigation of fractures and treatment as per orthopaedics.

Treatment
- Conservative: patient education, smoking cessation, alcohol cessation, nutrition, weighted exercise, FRAX score.
- Medical: oestrogen therapy in postmenopausal women (SERM/HRT), bisphosphonates, calcium and vitamin D supplements, RANKL inhibitors, e.g. denosumab.

Complications
- Pathological fractures (particularly the hip and spinal column).

MAP 8.4 **Metabolic Bone Disease** (*Continued*)

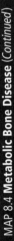

OSTEOPETROSIS

What is osteopetrosis?

This condition, also known as marble bone disease, occurs when osteoclasts do not function properly. As such bone is no longer resorbed. This means that bones are thick and fracture easily.

Causes

- Osteoclast dysfunction.

Signs and symptoms

- Asymptomatic.
- Hepatomegaly.
- Splenomegaly.
- Anaemia.

Investigations

- Bloods: FBC, U&Es, LFTs, TFTs, glucose, serum calcium, serum phosphate, alkaline phosphatase and PTH.
- Radiology: X-ray to assess fractures.

Treatment

- Conservative: patient education. Refer to physiotherapy.
- Medical: vitamin D, calcitriol, erythropoietin, corticosteroids, interferon-gamma, bone marrow transplant.

Complications

- Increased fracture risk.
- Neurological involvement due to nerve impingement.

PAGET'S DISEASE

What is Paget's disease?

This is a chronic remodelling disorder of bone that results in abnormal bone architecture.

Causes

The exact cause is unknown but it this thought to have a viral and genetic aetiology.

Signs and symptoms

- Asymptomatic.
- Bone pain.
- Pathological fracture.
- Hearing loss (if skull affected).

Investigations

- Bloods: FBC, U&Es, LFTs, TFTs, glucose, serum calcium, serum phosphate, alkaline phosphatase and PTH.
- Radiology: X-ray to assess fractures.

Treatment

- Conservative: patient education and management of complications.
- Medical: bisphosphonates such as zoledronate injections.

Complications

- Osteogenic sarcoma.
- Heart failure.
- Increased risk of renal calculi.

Map 8.4 Metabolic Bone Disease

Table 8.1 Biochemical Profiling in Different Metabolic Bone Diseases

TABLE 8.1 Biochemical Profiling in Different Metabolic Bone Diseases

Investigation	Osteoporosis	Osteomalacia	Osteopetrosis	Paget's disease
Serum calcium	Normal	↓	Normal	Normal
Serum phosphate	Normal	↓	Normal	Normal
Alkaline phosphatase	Normal	↑	↑	Varies with evolution of disease
PTH	Normal	↑	Normal	Normal

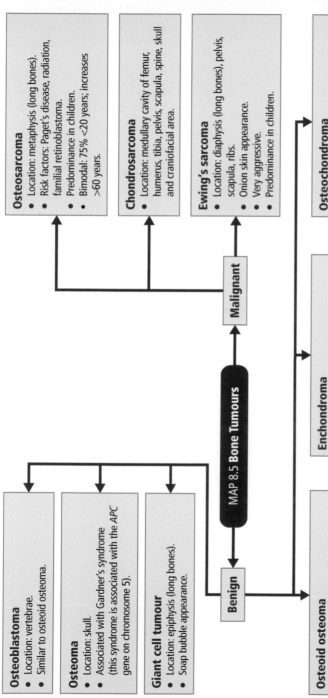

Osteoblastoma
- Location: vertebrae.
- Similar to osteoid osteoma.

Osteoma
- Location: skull.
- Associated with Gardner's syndrome (this syndrome is associated with the *APC* gene on chromosome 5).

Giant cell tumour
- Location: epiphysis (long bones).
- Soap bubble appearance.

Osteoid osteoma
- Location: femur and tibia, phalanges and vertebrae.
- Intracortical lesion best differentiated on CT.
- Nidus.

Benign

MAP 8.5 **Bone Tumours**

Malignant

Osteosarcoma
- Location: metaphysis (long bones).
- Risk factors: Paget's disease, radiation, familial retinoblastoma.
- Predominance in children.
- Bimodal: 75% <20 years; increases >60 years.

Chondrosarcoma
- Location: medullary cavity of femur, humerus, tibia, pelvis, scapula, spine, skull and craniofacial area.

Ewing's sarcoma
- Location: diaphysis (long bones), pelvis, scapula, ribs.
- Onion skin appearance.
- Very aggressive.
- Predominance in children.

Osteochondroma
- Location: metaphysis (long bones).
- Most common benign bone lesion.

Enchondroma
- Location: intramedullary bone.
- Cartilaginous neoplasm.
- Seen in phalanges.

Map 8.5 Bone Tumours

MAP 8.6 Systemic Lupus Erythematosus (SLE)

What is systemic lupus erythematosus (SLE)?

This is a multisystemic autoimmune disease that usually affects females of childbearing age.

Causes

The exact cause is unknown. However, an increased incidence is associated with HLA-B8, -DR2 and -DR3 as well as deficiencies in aspects of the complement pathway, e.g. C2 and C4. Criteria for diagnosing SLE have been revised as follows:

≥4/11 is diagnostic. Remember these as **I AM PORN HSD**.

- **I**mmunological disorder.
- **A**NA positive.
- **M**alar rash.
- **P**hotosensitivity.
- **O**ral ulcers.
- **R**enal disorder.
- **N**onerosive arthritis, **N**eurological disorder.
- **H**aematological disorder.
- **S**erositis.
- **D**iscoid rash.

Investigations

- Bloods: FBC, U&Es, LFTs, TFTs, glucose, CRP, ESR.
- Specific immune blood tests: antinuclear antibody (ANA). Anti-Smith antibodies and anti-double-stranded DNA. Other autoantibodies that may be seen are anti-smooth muscle, anti-Ro, anti-La, rheumatoid factor.
- Low complement levels.
- False-positive syphilis tests.
- ECG.
- Pulmonary function tests.

MAP 8.6 **Systemic Lupus Erythematosus (SLE)**

Treatment

- Conservative: patient education. Advise patient about sun protection and encourage smoking cessation. Assess psychological impact of disease.
- Medical: based on discussions with their rheumatologist.
  - Analgesia for joint pain.
  - Steroid therapy.
  - Classic immunosuppressants, e.g. cyclophosphamide, mycophenolate mofetil, methotrexate, azathioprine, hydroxychloroquine, leflunomide, cyclosporin, tacrolimus.
  - Monoclonal antibodies, e.g. rituximab.
  - Anti-interferon (IFN)-alpha monoclonal antibody, e.g. sifalimumab, rontalizumab.
  - Anti-malaria medications, e.g. hydroxychloroquine.

Complications

- Increased risk of atherosclerosis.
- Increased risk of stroke.
- Increased risk of myocardial infarction.
- Risk of lupus nephritis.
- Increased risk of other autoimmune conditions.

Signs and symptoms

- Eyes: vasculitis, conjunctivitis, episcleritis.
- Skin: malar butterfly rash, photosensitivity, Raynaud's phenomenon.
- Lungs: pulmonary fibrosis, pleurisy, effusion, pneumonitis.
- Heart: pericarditis, myocarditis.
- Kidneys: glomerulonephritis, proteinuria, nephrotic syndrome.
- MSK: small joint arthralgia, erosive arthritis, Jaccoud's arthropathy.

MAP 8.6 Systemic Lupus Erythematosus (SLE)

Map 8.7 Antiphospholipid Syndrome

What is antiphospholipid syndrome (APS)?

Also known as Hughes syndrome, this is an immune disorder that results in increased risk of blood clot formation.

Causes

APS may be primary (in the absence of evidence of autoimmune disease) or secondary (in the presence of other autoimmune disease, e.g. SLE). There is an association with HLA-DR7, -DR4, -DRw53 and -DQw7 and C4. Some infections such as HIV, *Borrelia burgdorferi* and *Treponema* have been associated with antiphospholipid antibody (APLA) formation.

Signs and symptoms

- Can be very mild and asymptomatic.
- Arterial +/− venous thrombosis affecting any organ.
- Morbidity related to pregnancy – miscarriage, intrauterine growth restriction, HELLP syndrome.
- Livedo reticularis.
- Mitral/aortic valve disease – regurgitation or stenosis.
- Stroke.
- Blindness.
- DVT/PE.

Treatment

- Conservative: patient education, cardiovascular risk assessment and modification of risk factors.
- Medical: requires discussion with rheumatologist/haematologist and may depend on patient factors such as age, if female and trying to become pregnant, or whether they have had multiple episodes of clot formation. Options include aspirin/clopidogrel for milder cases. For more severe cases drugs such as warfarin (with INR monitoring), apixaban, rivaroxaban and dabigatran may be considered.

Mechanism of action of drugs

- Aspirin: inhibits COX1 and COX2 enzymes in the arachidonic acid pathway, thereby reduces inflammatory prostaglandins.
- Clopidogrel: ADP receptor antagonist.
- Warfarin: vitamin K antagonist therefore inhibits factors II, VII, IX and X as well as proteins C and S.
- Apixaban: inhibits factor Xa.
- Rivaroxaban: inhibits factor Xa (prothrombinase complex).
- Dabigatran: directly inhibits thrombin (IIa).

MAP 8.7 Antiphospholipid Syndrome (APS)

Investigations

Blood tests include enzyme-linked immunosorbent assay (ELISA) and functional assays:

- Anticardiolipin antibodies IgG or IgM (ELISA).
- Anti-β_2-glycoprotein-I antibodies IgG or IgM (ELISA).
- Lupus anticoagulants (functional assays).

The revised Sapporo classification criteria for APS require at least one laboratory and one clinical criterion to be met.

Clinical criteria:

- Vascular thrombosis: ≥1 arterial, venous or small vessel thrombosis.
- Pregnancy morbidity.
  - ≥1 fetal death (at or beyond the 10th week of gestation).
  - ≥1 premature birth before the 34th week of gestation because of eclampsia, severe pre-eclampsia or placental insufficiency.
  - ≥3 consecutive (pre-)embryonic losses (before the 10th week of gestation).

Laboratory criteria:

- Lupus anticoagulant positivity on ≥2 occasions at least 12 weeks apart.
- Anticardiolipin antibody (IgG and/or IgM) in medium or high titre (i.e. >40, or above the 99th percentile), on two or more occasions at least 12 weeks apart.
- Anti-β_2-glycoprotein-I antibody (IgG and/or IgM) in medium or high titre (i.e. above the 99th percentile) on two or more occasions at least 12 weeks apart.

Complications

- DVT.
- Pulmonary embolism.
- Risks of lifelong anticoagulation.
- End organ damage for vessel occlusion, e.g. myocardial infarction, stroke.
- Cardiac valve disease.
- Pregnancy morbidity.
- Catastrophic antiphospholipid syndrome (CAPS). This is life threatening and has four criteria for diagnosis:
  - Involvement of three or more organ systems.
  - Manifestations developing simultaneously or within less than 1 week.
  - Histopathological confirmation of small-vessel occlusion in at least one organ/tissue.
  - Laboratory confirmation of the presence of antiphospholipid antibody.

Map 8.7 Antiphospholipid Syndrome

Map 8.8 Systemic Sclerosis and Scleroderma

What is systemic sclerosis and scleroderma?

This is a rare autoimmune condition that results in the thickening/hardening (sclerosis) of collagen in the skin (scleroderma) and internal organs (systemic sclerosis). It is more common in females.

MAP 8.8 **Systemic Sclerosis and Scleroderma**

Causes

The exact cause of the condition is unknown. *OX40L* gene polymorphism and the *IRF5* gene correlate with systemic scleroderma. Silica and certain organic solvents are recognised risk factors. Systemic sclerosis is associated with CREST syndrome (Calcinosis, Raynaud's disease, (o)Esophageal dysmotility, Sclerodactyly and Telangiectasia).

Signs and symptoms

- Scleroderma: morphoea, linear scleroderma.
- Systemic sclerosis:
  ○ Facial features – beaked nose/small mouth.
  ○ Raynaud's disease.
  ○ Heart – pericarditis, myocardial fibrosis, restrictive cardiomyopathy.
  ○ Lungs – pulmonary fibrosis.
  ○ GI system – GORD, oesophagitis.
  ○ Nervous system – peripheral neuropathy.
  ○ Renal system – acute or chronic kidney injury.

Investigations

To diagnose the condition and to look for complications.

- Blood tests: FBC, U&Es, LFTS, glucose, HbA1c, CRP and ESR, BNP (if heart failure expected).
- Autoantibodies: anti-centromere and anti-scl70/anti-topoisomerase antibodies, anti-RNA polymerase, rheumatoid factor.

Test looking for involved organs:

- Transthoracic echocardiography/ECG.
- CXR/hand X-ray.
- Diffusing capacity of the lung for carbon monoxide (DLCO) and spirometry.
- Oesophageal manometry/OGD.
- Urinalysis.

Treatment

- There is no curative treatment for this condition. Therefore, management aims at symptomatic control and slowing disease progression.
- Conservative: patient education. Yearly follow-up regarding NT-pro-BNP dosage, spirometry and DLCO, transthoracic echocardiography and urinalysis.
- Medical:
  ○ Localised scleroderma: topical corticosteroids for plaque morphea. Generalised morphea may require combination therapy with systemic steroids and methotrexate +/– phototherapy.
  ○ Raynaud's phenomenon: avoid cold weather triggers. Vasodilators, e.g. nifedipine.
  ○ Oesophageal symptoms: PPI, OGD +/– dilation for strictures.
  ○ Hypertension: as per NICE guidelines (see Map 1.6).
  ○ Immunosuppressive therapy is to be discussed with a rheumatologist but is generally reserved for diffuse systemic sclerosis.

MAP 8.9 **Sjögren's Syndrome**

What is Sjögren's syndrome?

This is an autoimmune disorder of the lacrimal and salivary glands. Up to 50% of these patients develop extra-glandular autoimmune involvement, e.g. the joints, skin, GI tract and renal system. Sjögren's syndrome may be associated with other autoimmune conditions such as SLE and RA. It is more common in females.

Causes

The exact cause of the condition is unknown. HLA-DQA and -DQB are associated with an increased risk of the condition. There is an association with non-Hodgkin's B cell lymphoma.

Signs and symptoms

- Eyes: grittiness, photosensitivity, keratoconjunctivitis sicca.
- GI system: xerostomia, mouth ulcers, non-tender enlargement of the parotid glands/submandibular glands.
- Arthralgia/polyarthritis.
- Raynaud's phenomenon.

Investigations

Bloods: FBC, U&Es, LFTs, CRP, ESR. Autoantibodies: ANA, anti-Ro, rheumatoid factor. Schirmer's test: measures tear production. Referral to ophthalmologist for a slit-lamp exam.

Treatment

- Conservative: patient education.
- Medical:
  - Eyes: artificial tears, eye drops.
  - Mouth: good oral hygiene, chewing gum, saliva substitutes, medications that increase saliva flow, e.g. pilocarpine.
  - Immunosuppressants to be discussed with rheumatologist, e.g. DMARDs (methotrexate, azathioprine).
  - Corticosteroids may be used in acute flares.

Complications

- Reduced visual acuity.
- Increase in oral yeast infections.
- Kidney dysfunction.
- Liver dysfunction.
- Increased risk of lymphoma and multiple myeloma.

Map 8.9 Sjögren's Syndrome

MAP 8.10 Marfan's Syndrome

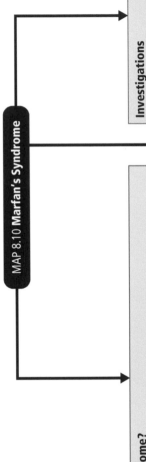

Investigations

This is a clinical diagnosis. Investigations involve cardiovascular and aneurysm assessment.

- CVS: bloods – FBC, U&Es, LFTs, HbA1c, cholesterol levels. ECG, transthoracic ECHO + follow-up.
- Ophthalmology referral for slit-lamp examination/assessment of lens dislocation.

What is Marfan's syndrome?

This is an inherited connective disorder with an incidence between 1 in 3,000 and 1 in 5,000.

Causes

Autosomal dominant inheritance resulting from mutations in the *FBN1* gene on chromosome 15, which codes for the glycoprotein fibrillin. Fibrillin is the main constituent of elastic fibres.

Signs and symptoms

- Cardiovascular system: aortic root disease, leading to aortic regurgitation, aneurysmal dilatation and dissection. Mitral valve prolapse and regurgitation.
- MSK: high arched palate, arachnodactyly, scoliosis, pectus excavatum.
- Ocular: upward lens dislocation.

The Ghent diagnostic criteria for Marfan's syndrome are outlined below:

System	Major criteria	Minor criteria
Family history	Independent diagnosis in parent, child or sibling	None
Genetics	Mutation *FBN1*	None
Cardiovascular	Aortic root dilatation, dissection of ascending aorta	Mitral valve prolapse, calcification of the mitral valve (<40 years), dilatation of the pulmonary artery, dilatation/ dissection of descending aorta
Ocular	Ectopia lentis	Two needed of the following: flat cornea, elongated globe, myopia
Skeletal	At least four of the following: pectus excavatum needing surgery, pectus carinatum, pes planus, positive wrist or thumb sign, scoliosis >20° or spondylolisthesis, armspan:height ratio >1.05, protrusio acetabulae, diminished extension elbows (<170°)	For the skeletal system to be involved, two to three major or one major and two minor signs should be present: moderate pectus excavatum, high arched palate, typical facial features and joint hypermobility
Pulmonary		Spontaneous pneumothorax, apical bulla
Skin		Striae, recurrent or incisional herniae
Central nervous system	Lumbosacral dural ectasia	

Treatment

- Conservative: patient education, genetic counselling, annual ECHO, orthopaedic and ophthalmology referrals may be required.
- Medical: beta-blockers.
- Surgical: elective aortic root repair.

Complications

- Cardiovascular complications: aortic aneurysm and dissection, mitral valve prolapse, mitral regurgitation, aortic regurgitation.
- Ophthalmic complications: lens subluxation (ectopia lentis), cataract, glaucoma and retinal detachment.
- Spontaneous pneumothorax.
- Inguinal hernias.
- Scoliosis.

Map 8.10 Marfan's Syndrome

Map 8.11 Polymyalgia Rheumatica

What is polymyalgia rheumatica (PMR)?

This is a rheumatic disorder characterised by pain and stiffness around the shoulders, neck and pelvic girdle. It is associated with temporal arteritis. It is more common in females and those >50 years old.

MAP 8.11 **Polymyalgia Rheumatica**

Investigations

- Bloods: FBC (anaemia of chronic disease), U&Es, LFTs (alkaline phosphatase is occasionally elevated), ESR elevated, CRP elevated.
- Serological tests: antinuclear antibody (ANA), rheumatoid factor (RF) and anti-citrullinated protein antibodies (anti-CCP) are negative.

USS/MRI: assessment of subacromial/subdeltoid bursitis, long head of biceps tenosynovitis and glenohumeral synovitis. MRI is more sensitive for hip and pelvic girdle disease.

Causes

The exact cause of this condition is unknown. The *HLA-DRB1*04* allele correlates most frequently with familial aggregation of PMR.

Signs and symptoms

- Pain, stiffness and arthralgia of gradual onset around the neck, shoulders and pelvic girdle, i.e. glenohumeral and hip joints, and in the subacromial, subdeltoid and trochanteric bursae. This is perceived to be symmetrical and can be associated with restricted range of movement.
- Systemic features such as fatigue, weight loss and anorexia.
- Low grade fever.
- Temporal arteritis (see Map 8.12).

Treatment

- Conservative: includes modifying risk factors for osteoporosis (see Map 8.4) and patient education.
- Medical: to be discussed with rheumatologist but typically involves low dose steroids, medications to prevent the risk of osteoporosis, e.g. vitamin D and calcium supplementation/bisphosphonate prophylaxis and PPI to protect the stomach.

Complications

- Temporal (giant cell) arteritis, which may result in blindness.
- Risk of long-term steroid use, which can be remembered by the **CUSHINGOID** mnemonic:
  - **C**ataracts.
  - **U**lcers.
  - **S**kin: striae, thinning, bruising.
  - **H**ypertension/hirsutism/hyperglycaemia.
  - **I**nfections.
  - **N**ecrosis, avascular necrosis of the femoral head.
  - **G**lycosuria.
  - **O**steoporosis, obesity.
  - **I**mmunosuppression.
  - **D**iabetes.

2012 Provisional classification criteria for polymyalgia rheumatica: a European League Against Rheumatism/American College of Rheumatology collaborative initiative

'Patients aged 50 years or older with bilateral shoulder aching and abnormal C-reactive protein concentrations or ESR, plus at least four points (without ultrasonography) or five points or more (with ultrasonography) from:

- Morning stiffness in excess of 45 minutes duration (two points).
- Hip pain or restricted range of motion (one point).
- Absence of rheumatoid factor or anti-citrullinated protein antibodies (two points).
- Absence of other joint involvement (one point).
- If ultrasonography is available, at least one shoulder with subdeltoid bursitis, biceps tenosynovitis or glenohumeral synovitis (either posterior or axillary); and at least one hip with synovitis or trochanteric bursitis (one point).
- If ultrasonography is available, both shoulders with subdeltoid bursitis, biceps tenosynovitis, or glenohumeral synovitis (one point).'

Map 8.11 Polymyalgia Rheumatica

MAP 8.12 Temporal (Giant Cell) Arteritis

What is temporal (giant cell) arteritis?

This is a chronic vasculitis characterised by granulomatous inflammation in the walls of medium and large arteries. It typically affects people over 50 years of age and has an incidence of 2.2 per 10,000.

Causes

The exact cause is unknown. There is an association with Toll-like receptor 4 gene polymorphism, *HLA-DRB1*04 and HLA Class II genes.
Risk factors include advancing age and Scandinavian ancestry.

Signs and symptoms

- New-onset headache that is usually unilateral in the temporal area.
- Temporal artery tenderness, thickening or nodularity.
- Visual disturbance, e.g. vision loss, decreased visual acuity, diplopia.
- Scalp tenderness.
- Intermittent jaw claudication.
- Systemic features, e.g. fever, fatigue, anorexia, weight loss.
- Features of polymyalgia rheumatica.
- Neurological features, e.g. stroke.
- Bruits.
- Blood pressure difference between arms.
- Intermittent limb claudication.

Investigations

- Blood tests: elevated ESR.
- Temporal artery biopsy.

The American College of Rheumatology (ACR) has developed a set of criteria for diagnosing temporal arteritis. Three of the five criteria must be present to make the diagnosis:

- Age greater than or equal to 50 at the onset of symptoms.
- New headache.
- Temporal artery abnormalities such as tenderness of the superficial artery or decreased pulsation.
- ESR greater than or equal to 50 mm/h.
- Abnormal artery biopsy, including vasculitis, a predominance of mononuclear cell infiltration or granulomatous inflammation, or multinucleated giant cells.

Treatment

- Conservative: patient education, factors and comorbidities relevant to steroid therapy (e.g. diabetes, hypertension, glaucoma, peptic ulcer and bone fracture risk). Consideration of preventive measures (e.g. vitamin D and calcium supplements, bisphosphonates and PPI).
- Medical: temporal arteritis is a medical emergency.
  - If the patient has any visual disturbances, then they must immediately be referred for urgent ophthalmology assessment.
  - Patients must be discussed with a rheumatology specialist urgently. Typically, glucocorticoid therapy is recommended. NICE recommends a dose of 40–60 mg PO prednisolone daily.

Complications

- Blindness.
- Large artery complications, e.g. aortic aneurysm, aortic dissection and large artery stenosis.
- Cardiovascular disease, e.g. stroke.
- Complications associated with steroid use.

Map 8.12 Temporal (Giant Cell) Arteritis

Map 8.13 Takayasu's Arteritis

What is Takayasu's arteritis?

This is a systemic inflammatory condition that is characterised by damage to the large and medium arteries as well as their branches. Typically affects young females and is more common in those of Asian descent.

Investigations

- Blood tests: FBC, U&Es, LFTs, CRP, ESR, glucose, lipid profile, cholesterol.
- Radiology: CTA (visualisation of vessel wall thickening and luminal narrowing). MRA may also be used (provides multiplanar imaging without ionising radiation).

Ishikawa clinical classification of Takayasu's arteritis

Group	Clinical features
Group I	Uncomplicated disease, with or without pulmonary artery involvement
Group IIA	Mild/moderate single complication together with uncomplicated disease
Group IIB	Severe single complication together with uncomplicated disease
Group III	Two or more complications together with uncomplicated disease

MAP 8.13 Takayasu's Arteritis

Causes

The exact aetiology is unknown.

Signs and symptoms

- Systemic features, e.g. myalgia, weight loss, fatigue, anorexia.
- Pulselessness (secondary to arterial insufficiencies).
- Hypertension.
- Neurological manifestations, e.g. secondary to carotid artery occlusion, upper limb claudication.
- Debilitating upper or lower extremity ischaemia, which lead to diminished or absent pulses +/− ischaemic ulceration/gangrene.
- Vascular bruit.

Treatment

- Conservative: patient education, modification of cardiovascular risk factors.
- Medical: corticosteroids.

Complications

- Takayasu's retinopathy.
- Secondary hypertension.
- Aortic regurgitation.
- Aneurysm formation.
- Limb ischaemia.
- Stroke.
- Heart failure.

What is Henoch–Schönlein purpura?

This is an IgA-mediated immune vasculitis involving the small vessels of the joints, kidneys, gastrointestinal (GI) tract and skin. More infrequently it can affect the central nervous system and lungs. It affects males more than females, and is more common in children.

Causes

The exact cause is unknown. In most patients there are reports of a preceding upper respiratory tract infection. The following organisms have been implicated: group A *Streptococcus*, Coxsackievirus, hepatitis A, hepatitis B, *Mycoplasma*, parvovirus B19, *Campylobacter*, varicella and adenoviruses. IgA plays a significant role.

Signs and symptoms

- Systemic features: fevers, fatigue.
- Skin: non-pruritic, palpable purpura and petechiae typically over the buttock and lower extremities.
- GI tract: abdominal pain, nausea, vomiting, melaena, haematemesis.
- Renal: haematuria, proteinuria (nephrotic syndrome).
- MSK: arthralgia.
- CNS: rarely involved but may have headaches, seizures and coma.

MAP 8.14 Henoch–Schönlein Purpura

Investigations

- There is no specific test for Henoch–Schönlein purpura.
- Bloods: FBC, U&E, LFTs, CRP, IgA.
- Urinalysis

Treatment

- There is no specific treatment. The foundation of management is symptomatic support unless there is renal involvement which will require specialist renal physician support.
- Medical: supportive care with IV fluids for rehydration, analgesia, wound care. If Henoch–Schönlein purpura nephritis, seek renal advice and treatment may involve corticosteroids, plasma exchange and immunosuppressants

Complications

- Renal: acute kidney injury, chronic kidney injury, proteinuria, haematuria, nephrotic syndrome.
- GI tract: GI bleeding, intussusception, bowel perforation/infarction.
- CNS: seizures, coma.
- Respiratory: pleural effusion, pulmonary haemorrhage.

Map 8.14 Henoch–Schönlein Purpura

Map 8.15 Raynaud's Disease and Phenomenon

What are Raynaud's disease and phenomenon?

In this condition there is a transient and peripheral vasoconstrictive response of the digital arteries and cutaneous arterioles to cold temperatures +/– emotional stress. The condition may be either primary or secondary. It is more common in women than men and typically presents in young individuals.

Causes

- Primary Raynaud's disease occurs in the absence of other pathology.
- Secondary Raynaud's is associated with the following:
  - Connective tissue disease: SLE, scleroderma and Sjögren's syndrome.
  - Infections: parvovirus B19, cytomegalovirus, hepatitis B and hepatitis C.
  - Drugs: interferon-alpha and -beta, ciclosporin, non-selective beta-blockers.
  - Occupational exposure: hand–arm vibration syndrome (vibrating machinery).

Symptoms

Symmetrical changing from white to blue to red typically affecting one finger first and then becoming more generalised. It affects the hands more than the feet.

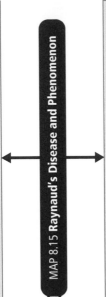

MAP 8.15 **Raynaud's Disease and Phenomenon**

Investigations

- There is no specific test for Raynaud's disease.
- It is important to differentiate between primary and secondary Raynaud's disease and therefore one may wish to perform tests looking for underlying connective tissue disorders.
- These may include FBC, ESR and ANA, as well as other tests outlined in previous mind maps.

Management

- Conservative: patient education, Raynaud Condition Score (RCS), smoking cessation, regular exercise, minimise stress if trigger, aim to keep the whole body warm, consider gloves and warm footwear, avoid cold environments.
- Medical: urgent admission if patient has digit ischaemia. Referral to rheumatology especially if underlying connective tissue disorder suspected. Consider a trial of nifedipine as prophylaxis.

Chapter Nine **Infectious Disease**

Map 9.1 Malaria

What is malaria?

This is an infectious disease caused by parasitic *Plasmodium*, which is spread by the female *Anopheles* mosquito.

Causes

- *Plasmodium falciparum*: most severe form. Causes cerebral malaria.
- *P. ovale*: may lie dormant within the liver as hypnozoites.
- *P. vivax*: may lie dormant within the liver as hypnozoites.
- *P. malariae*.
- *P. knowlesi*: very rare.

Signs and symptoms

- Fatigue.
- Night sweats.
- Flu-like symptoms.
- Diarrhoea.
- Nausea.
- Vomiting.
- Anaemia.
- Splenomegaly.
- Seizures (cerebral malaria or secondary to fever).

Treatment

- Conservative; patient education. Prevention of disease, e.g. mosquito nets and repellent sprays.
- Medical: prophylactic and therapeutic. Treatment is dependent on *Plasmodium* species:
  - Inhibit haem polymerase:
    - Chloroquine.
    - Quinine.
  - Blood schizonticide:
    - Mefloquine.
    - Primaquine.
    - Malarone.
  - Inhibits plasmodial protein synthesis: doxycycline.
  - Inhibits dihydrofolate reductase: pyrimethamine.
  - Inhibits falciparum sarcoplasmic–endoplasmic reticulum calcium ATPase: artemether (always used with lumefantrine).
  - Inhibits haem metabolism: lumefantrine.
- Surgical: splenectomy, if indicated.

Investigations

- Bloods: FBC, U&Es, creatinine, LFTs, ESR, CRP.
- Blood film.
- Real-time PCR.
- Antigen detection kits.

Complications

- Cerebral malaria.
- Anaemia.
- Hepatic failure.
- Splenomegaly.
- Shock.
- Acute kidney injury.
- Dehydration.
- Acute respiratory distress syndrome (ARDS).

MAP 9.1 **Malaria**

FIGURE 9.1 **Malaria Lifecycle**

Infected mosquito bites human host

Sporozoites enter the circulatory system

The sporozoites travel in the blood to the liver where they infect hepatocytes

Within the hepatocyte the sporozoites mature into schizonts, which produce many merozoites. *P. vivax* has an additional dormant stage where the sporozoites become hypnozoites

These merozoites replicate until their vast numbers eventually rupture the hepatocytes. In doing this the merozoites enter the bloodstream and infect red blood cells

Within the red blood cells merozoites continue to replicate until the red blood cells rupture

Some of these red blood cells become gametocytes, which remain in the blood for a few days. During this time the gametocytes may be transferred to a mosquito that feeds on this infected human

Within the mosquito the gametocytes turn into sporozoites and the mosquito is now a vector of disease

Malaria lifecycle: transmitted by female *Anopheles* mosquito

Figure 9.1 Malaria Lifecycle

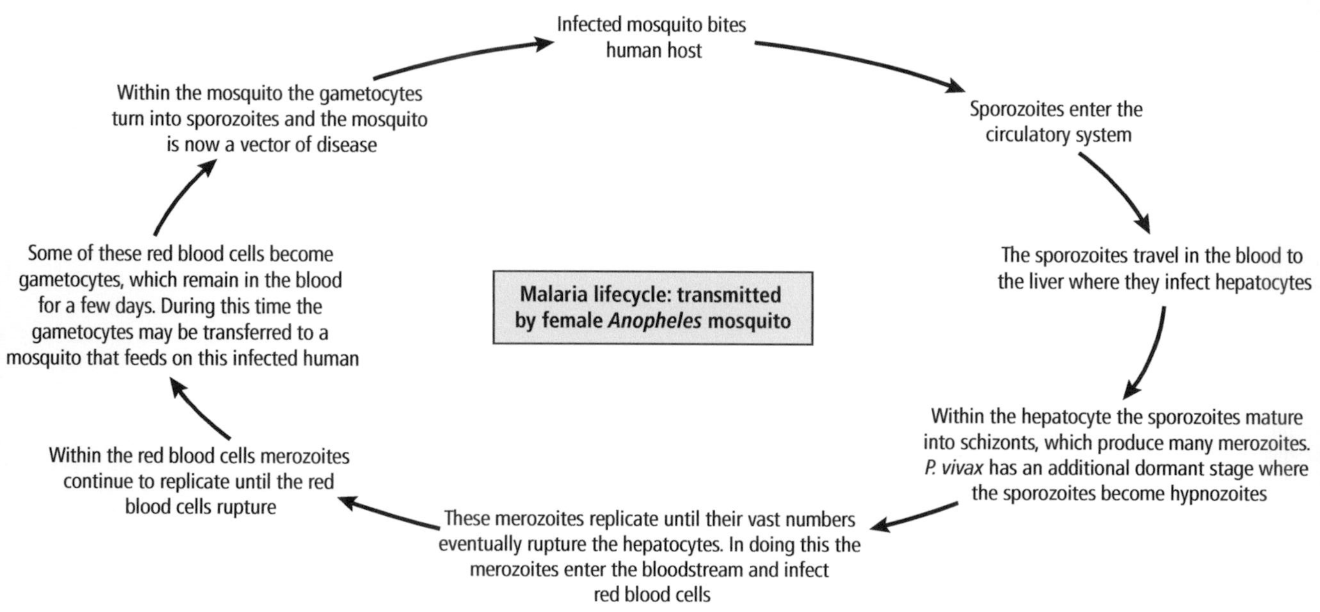

Map 9.2 Tuberculosis (TB)

What is TB?

TB is a granulomatous disease that may affect any organ, but most commonly affects the lungs since it is transmitted via aerosol droplets.

Causes

Mycobacterium tuberculosis (acid-fast bacillus).

Pathophysiology

- Primary pulmonary TB:
  ○ Initial TB infection.
  ○ Ghon focus formation in upper lobes.
  ○ Hilar lymphadenopathy.
- Secondary pulmonary TB:
  ○ Occurs after primary infection.
  ○ Dormant TB is reactivated.
  ○ Fibrocaseous lesions.
- Other forms of TB:
  ○ Miliary.
  ○ Genitourinary.
  ○ Bone, e.g. Pott's disease of the spine.
  ○ Peritoneal.
  ○ Meningitis.

Treatment

- Conservative: patient education, especially the importance of complying with medical therapy.
- Medical – remember **RIPE**:
  ○ **R**ifampicin.
  ○ **I**soniazid.
  ○ **P**yrazinamide.
  ○ **E**thambutol.

  Other drugs that may be used in therapy include: streptomycin, quinolones, amikacin and capreomycin.

- Surgical: depends on location, e.g. for pulmonary TB consider lobectomy.

Investigations

- Sputum culture:
  Ogawa/Löwenstein–Jensen medium.
- Sputum stain: Ziehl–Neelsen stain.
- Transbronchial biopsy: granulomas are diagnostic.
- Pleural fluid analysis and biopsy.
- Radiology: X-ray for infiltrates and cavitations. Lesions described as millet seeds in miliary TB.

Signs and symptoms

- Cough.
- Haemoptysis.
- Weight loss.
- Night sweats.
- Fever.

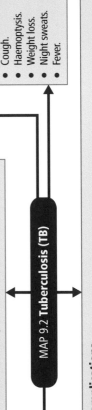

MAP 9.2 **Tuberculosis (TB)**

Complications

- Dissemination to other organs.
- Death.
- Side effects of anti-TB drugs
  ○ Rifampicin – discoloured secretions, hepatotoxicity, gastrointestinal upset, antibiotic resistance.
  ○ Isoniazid – vitamin B_6 deficiency, which can lead to peripheral neuropathy (therefore give with pyridoxine), hepatotoxicity, seborrhoeic dermatitis, confusion, seizures.
  ○ Pyrazinamide – hepatotoxicity.
  ○ Ethambutol – retrobulbar neuritis.

FIGURE 9.2 **Mode of Infection of Pulmonary TB**

Mode of infection

Droplets inhaled

Bacteria colonise alveoli

Bacteria engulfed by macrophages

Multiplication of bacteria within macrophages

Granulomas form around *M. tuberculosis* (caseous necrosis)

Immunocompetent patients – caseous necrosis produces conditions that decrease the growth of bacteria, e.g. lowered oxygen and pH levels

Latency

Non-immunocompetent patients – granuloma formation does not contain bacteria

Liquefaction of necrotic tissue

Coughing of infectious droplets since the liquified necrotic tissue drains into the bronchus

Figure 9.2 Mode of Infection of Pulmonary TB

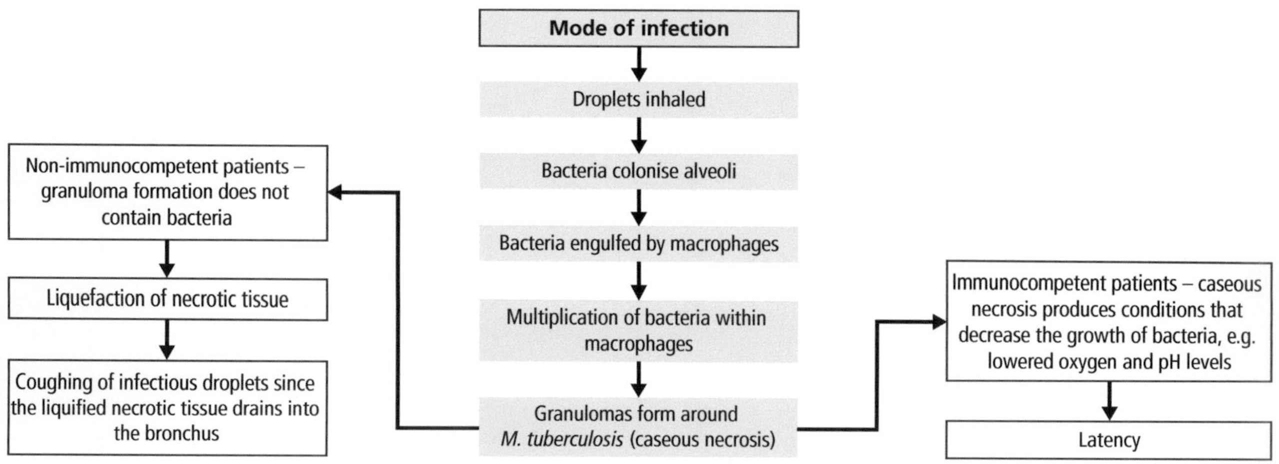

Map 9.3 Human Herpes Virus (HHV)

MAP 9.3 Human Herpes Virus (HHV)

HHV-1
- Herpes labialis.

Note
HHV-1 and HHV-2 may affect both the mouth and the genitals.

HHV-2
- Herpes genitalis.

Investigations
A clinical diagnosis, which may be confirmed by culturing the virus and by immunofluorescence.

Treatment
- Conservative: patient education and methods to reduce spread.
- Medical: antiviral medications, e.g. aciclovir and famciclovir.

HHV-8
- Kaposi's sarcoma (associated with HIV).

HHV-7
- Belongs to the subfamily betaherpesvirinae.
- It is closely related to HHV-6.

HHV-6
- Roseola infantum.

Cytomegalovirus (HHV-5)
- Mononucleosis (negative Monospot test).
- Typically seen in immunocompromised patients.
- Transmitted via sexual contact, saliva, urine, transplant, transfusion and congenitally.

Epstein–Barr virus (HHV-4)
- Infectious mononucleosis – 'kissing disease' (positive Monospot test).
- Associated with Burkitt's lymphoma.
- Associated with nasopharyngeal carcinoma.
- Transmitted via droplet infection and saliva.

Varicella-zoster virus (HHV-3)
- Chickenpox.
- Shingles.

Map 9.3 Human Herpes Virus (HHV)

Map 9.4 Human Immunodeficiency Virus (HIV)

What is HIV?

HIV is an RNA retrovirus of the lentivirus genus.
This virus causes acquired immunodeficiency syndrome (AIDS).

Causes

There are two types of HIV:

1 HIV-1:
- Type M: A–J prevalent in Europe, America, Australia and sub-Saharan Africa.
- Type O: mainly in Cameroon.

2 HIV-2: predominantly confined to West Africa.

Transmission

- Unprotected sexual intercourse.
- Shared contaminated needles.
- Contaminated blood transfusions.
- Vertical transmission from mother to child.
The virus crosses the placenta and is transmitted through breast milk.

Investigations

- Bloods: FBC, U&Es, LFTs, lipids, glucose, HLA-B*5701 status, lymphocyte subsets.
- HIV specific:
  ○ Enzyme-linked immunosorbent assay (ELISA).
  ○ Western blot test.
  ○ Immunofluorescence assay (IFA).
  ○ Nucleic acid testing.
- Virology screen: HIV antibody, HIV viral load, HIV genotype, hepatitis serology, cytomegalovirus (CMV) antibody, syphilis screen.
- Other infection, e.g. tuberculosis if indicated.
- Baseline tests in 'exposure groups'.
  ○ All exposures:
    ■ Creatinine (and eGFR).
    ■ Alanine transaminase.
    ■ HIV-1 Ag/Ab.
    ■ If not known to be vaccinated with documented HepBsAb >10 IU: hepatitis B serology (HepBsAg, HepBsAb, HepBcAb).
  ○ Sexual exposure: as for 'all exposures', plus chlamydia, gonorrhoea and syphilis testing. Hep C screening in men who have sex with men and others at risk of hepatitis C.

Complications

- Increased risk of opportunistic infections:
  ○ Toxoplasmosis.
  ○ CMV, e.g. retinitis.
  ○ *Pneumocystis jiroveci* pneumonia.
  ○ Cryptococcal meningitis.
  ○ *Mycobacterium avium* complex.
  ○ *Candida*.
  ○ Aspergillosis.
- Increased risk of malignancies:
  ○ Kaposi's sarcoma.
  ○ Non-Hodgkin's lymphoma.
  ○ Cervical cancer.
  ○ Anal cancer.

MAP 9.4 **Human Immunodeficiency Virus (HIV)**

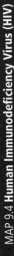

Treatment

- Conservative: patient education, transmission reduction advice, contact tracing, psychological support.
- Medical:
  - HIV post-exposure prophylaxis: the recommended first-line PEP regimen is tenofovir disoproxil 245 mg/emtricitabine 200 mg with raltegravir 1200 mg once daily for a minimum of 28 days. Final HIV testing is recommended at a minimum of 45 days after the PEP course is completed. If the 28-day course is completed, this is a minimum of 73 days (10.5 weeks) after exposure. For sexual exposures this can be performed at 12 weeks to align with syphilis testing.
  - Antiretroviral therapy (ART): this is recommended at any CD4 count. The current guidelines suggest using a) tenofovir plus emtricitabine, these 2 drugs come in a single pill (Truvada) PLUS b) 1 of the following 6 options: dolutegravir, elvitegravir boosted with cobicistat, raltegravir, atazanavir boosted with ritonavir, darunavir boosted with ritonavir, rilpivirine.

Stopping ART is not recommended as viral load rebounds quickly in almost everyone who stops ART, and the CD4 count drops. See BHIVA guidelines for more information (details in Appendix Two).

Infection process

- gp120 antigen on HIV binds to CD4$^+$ receptors on the T cell.
- This process produces a conformational change and the need to bind to a co-receptor: CCR5 or CXCR4.
- gp41 binds to the co-receptor.
- This binding causes 'six-helix bundle formation' and fusion of the viral and host membranes.
- Disintegration of the viral capsid occurs causing viral RNA to be released into the human cell.
- Double-stranded RNA is produced and this process is catalysed by viral reverse transcriptase.
- Double-stranded RNA is integrated into host DNA using integrase enzyme.
- Host cell now manufactures new virions by long terminal repeat sequences and genes *tat* and *rev*.

Genes required for viral replication

Remember PEG:
- *pol* : encodes reverse transcriptase and integrase.
- *env* : encodes envelope proteins, e.g. gp120.
- *gag* : encodes viral structural proteins.

Map 9.5 Sexually Transmitted Infections (STIs)

TRICHOMONAS VAGINALIS
What is Trichomonas vaginalis?
It is an anaerobic protozoon, which causes trichomoniasis. Symptoms include a fishy bubbly thin discharge and on speculum examination 'strawberry' cervix is visible.

Investigations
- Cervical smear.
- Rapid antigen testing.
- PCR technique.

Treatment
Metronidazole. Intravaginal clotrimazole during pregnancy.

Complications
- Increased risk of HIV infection
- Increased risk of cervical cancer.
- Increased risk of preterm delivery.

GARDNERELLA VAGINALIS
What is Gardnerella vaginalis?
This is a facultative anaerobic coccobacillus that causes bacterial vaginosis ('fishy odour' and grey discharge). N.B. This is NOT an STI but does cause vaginal discharge and, as such, is included in differential diagnosis with chlamydia and gonorrhoea.

Investigations
- Microscopy – clue cells observed.

Treatment
- Metronidazole or clindamycin.

Complications
- Rarely causes complications.

TREPONEMA PALLIDUM
What is Treponema pallidum?
This is a spirochaete that causes syphilis. Infection occurs in 3 stages:
1 Chancre: painless superficial ulceration.
2 Disseminated disease: systemic involvement, rash seen on palms and soles.
3 Cardiac and neurological involvement.

Investigations
- Venereal Disease Research Laboratory (VDRL) test.
- Rapid plasma regain (RPR) test.
- Treponema pallidum particle agglutination.
- Fluorescent treponemal antibody absorption (FTA) test.
- Treponema pallidum haemagglutination (TPHA) test.
- Treponema pallidum particle agglutination (TPPA) test.
- Treponemal enzyme immunoassay (EIA).

Treatment
- Procaine penicillin G, doxycycline, erythromycin, azithromycin.
- N.B. If the patient has neurosyphilis then give them prophylactic prednisolone to avoid the Jarisch–Herxheimer reaction. This reaction may occur after antibacterial treatment, which causes the death of the spirochaete and subsequent endotoxin release. Endotoxins cause the Jarisch–Herxheimer reaction.

MAP 9.5 **Sexually Transmitted Infections (STIs)**

Complications
- Gumma formation.
- Meningitis.
- Stroke.
- Heart valve damage.

NEISSERIA GONORRHOEAE
What is *Neisseria gonorrhoeae*?
This is a Gram-negative diplococcus that causes gonorrhoea.
It is sometimes asymptomatic or presents with discharge.

Investigations
- NAAT.
- Cultured on chocolate agar.

Treatment
- Azithromycin (single dose) and ceftriaxone (single dose).

Complications
- Pelvic inflammatory disease.
- Infertility.
- Dissemination of bacteria.

Remember 3Hs:
- Hepatitis see page 52.
- Herpes see page 188.
- HIV see page 190.

CHLAMYDIA TRACHOMATIS
What is *Chlamydia trachomatis*?
This is a Gram-negative bacterium that causes chlamydia.

Investigations
- *Chlamydia* cell culture.
- Nucleic acid amplification test (NAAT).
- Direct fluorescent antibody test (DFA).

Treatment
- Azithromycin (single dose) or doxycycline (for 7 days).

Complications
- Pelvic inflammatory disease.
- Urethritis.
- Infertility.
- Postpartum endometritis.

Map 9.5 Sexually Transmitted Infections (STIs)

Map 9.6 Bacterial Infections

Staphylococcal infections
Staphylococcus aureus causes:
- Skin infections.
- Osteomyelitis.
- Pneumonia.
- Endocarditis.
- Toxic shock syndrome.

Virulence factors – remember **SET**:
- **S**urface proteins for adherence.
- **E**nzymes.
- **T**oxins.

Grow in clusters.

Gram-positive bacteria stain blue and pink with Gram stain. This is retained when washed with ethanol and water.

Gram-negative bacteria do not retain Gram stain when washed with ethanol and acetone.

Diphtheria
- *Corynebacterium diphtheriae.*
- Rod shaped.
- Exotoxin causes damage to the heart and nerves.

Anthrax
Spore-forming bacillus.

Whooping cough
Bordetella pertussis, a coccobacillus.

Plague
Yersinia pestis.

***Pseudomonas* infection**
Pseudomonas aeruginosa is an opportunistic aerobic bacillus.

Neisserial infections
- *Neisseria meningitidis*: meningitis.
- *N. gonorrhoeae*: sexually transmitted infection (STI), see page 193.

Gram-negative

Gram-positive

MAP 9.6 **Bacterial Infections**

Granuloma inguinale

- *Klebsiella granulomatis*.
- An encapsulated coccobacillus.
- Causes ulcerative genital infection.

Chancroid

- *Haemophilus ducreyi*.
- Causes ulcerative genital infection.

Nocardia

- *Nocardia asteroides*.
- Aerobic.
- Grows in branched chains.
- Causes opportunistic respiratory infections with central nervous system involvement.

Listeriosis

- *Listeria monocytogenes*.
- Facultative intracellular bacillus.
- Causes meningitis in elderly and immunosuppressed people.

Streptococcal infections

- Facultative or obligate anaerobes.
- *Streptococcus pneumoniae*: acquired pneumonia, see page 29 and meningitis.
- Enterococci: urinary tract infection and endocarditis.

Virulence factors:

- Capsules, which resist phagocytosis.
- M protein, which inhibits the alternative pathway of the complement system.
- Pneumolysin, which destroys the membranes of host cells.

Grow in pairs or chains.

Map 9.6 Bacterial Infections

Map 9.7 Viral Infections

MAP 9.7 Viral Infections

TRANSIENT INFECTIONS

Rhinovirus
- Enterovirus.
- Causes the common cold.

Influenza
- RNA virus.
- Causes the flu.
- Classified into 3 types: A, B and C.

Polio virus
- Unencapsulated RNA enterovirus.

Measles
- RNA paramyxovirus.
- Host cells develop T cell-mediated immunity to control this viral infection.
- Rash is caused by hypersensitivity to the viral antigens within the skin.

Mumps
- Paramyxovirus.
- Causes inflammation of the parotid glands.
- Sometimes travels to central nervous system (CNS), pancreas and testes.

West Nile virus
- Arthropod virus of the flavivirus group.
- Invades the CNS causing meningitis and encephalitis.
- Seen in elderly and immunosuppressed people.

Chronic latent infections
- Human herpes virus (HHV): see page 188.
- Cytomegalovirus (CMV): see page 189.
- Varicella-zoster virus (VZV): see page 189.

Chronic productive infections
- Hepatitis virus, see page 52.

TRANSFORMING INFECTIONS

Human immunodeficiency virus (HIV)
See page 190.

Human papillomavirus (HPV)
This is associated with cervical cancer (this is because the HPV E6 and HPV E7 gene products dysregulate the cell cycle).

Epstein–Barr virus (EBV)
- Causes infectious mononucleosis.
- Usually self-limiting.
- Presents with fever and sore throat.
- Associated with Burkitt's lymphoma (t[8;14] translocation of c-MYC oncogene), see page 189.

MAP 9.8 **Vaccines**

DNA vaccines
- Potentially in the future.
- Usually a harmless virus which has a gene for a protective antigen spliced into it.
- This protective antigen is generated within the vaccine recipient and elicits an immune response.

Advantages:
- Plasmids are easily manufactured and do not replicate.
- DNA is stable and sequencing may be changed.
- Temperature extremes are resisted; therefore, it is easily transported and stored.
- Cheap.

Disadvantages:
- Plasmids could integrate into the host genome.
- Immunological tolerance.

Subunit
- E.g. hepatitis B, tetanus, diphtheria.
- This is a vaccine containing purified components of the virus.
- Example components include the surface antigen.

Continued overleaf

Map 9.8 Vaccines

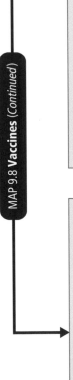

MAP 9.8 **Vaccines** (*Continued*)

Inactivated

- E.g. polio (Salk), rabies, hepatitis A, influenza.
- Preparations of the wild-type virus.
- The virus is non-pathogenic because of chemical treatment (e.g. with formalin).
- This chemical treatment cross-links viral proteins.

Advantages:
- Sufficient humoral immunity if boosters given.
- Good for immunosuppressed patients.
- No mutations of virus.
- Good for those living in tropical areas.

Disadvantages:
- Some do not increase immunity.
- Boosters are required.
- Expensive.
- Potential failure of viral inactivation process.
- Little local immunity.

Attenuated

- E.g. polio (Sabin), mumps, measles, rubella (MMR), varicella, rotavirus, yellow fever.
- Live virus particles grow in the vaccine recipient.
- However, these particles do not cause disease because the virus has been mutated to a form that is non-pathogenic, e.g. the virus tropism has been altered.

Advantages:
- Activates all phases of the immune system.
- It stimulates antibodies against multiple epitopes.
- Provides cheap and fast immunity.
- It has the potential to eliminate the wild-type virus from the community.
- Easily transported.

Disadvantages:
- If the mutation fails then the virus will revert to its virulent form.
- Potential spread of the mutated viral form.
- Do NOT give to immunocompromised patients.
- Not good for those living in tropical areas.

Map 10.1 Reproductive Hormones

OESTROGEN

Secreted by
• Ovaries and placenta.

Function
• Genital development.
• Breast development.
• Follicle growth.
• Endometrial growth.
• Upregulates oestrogen, LH and progesterone receptors.
• Inhibits FSH and LH through feedback mechanism.
• Stimulates prolactin secretion.
• Stimulates LH surge, which causes ovulation.
• Increases protein transport.

INHIBIN

Secreted by
• Sertoli cells.

Function
• Inhibits FSH.

PROGESTERONE

Secreted by
• Corpus luteum, placenta, adrenal cortex and testes.

Function
• Maintains pregnancy.
• Produces cervical mucus.
• Increases body temperature.
• Inhibits LH and FSH.
• Relaxes uterine smooth muscle.
• Downregulates oestrogen receptors.
• Increases endometrial gland secretion.
• Increases spiral artery development.
• Softens ligaments during pregnancy.

MAP 10.1 **Reproductive Hormones**

FOLLICLE-STIMULATING HORMONE (FSH)

Secreted by
- Anterior pituitary gland.

Function
- Stimulates Sertoli cells to produce androgen binding protein.
- Stimulates Sertoli cells to produce inhibin.

TESTOSTERONE

Secreted by
- Leydig cells of the testes and adrenal cortex.

Function
- Male secondary sexual characteristics.
- Penile and muscular development.
- Growth of seminal vesicles.
- Epiphyseal plate closure.
- Differentiation of vas deferens, seminal vesicles and epididymis.

LUTEINISING HORMONE (LH)

Secreted by
- Anterior pituitary gland.

Function
- Stimulates Leydig cells to produce testosterone.
- Surge causes ovulation.

Map 10.1 Reproductive Hormones

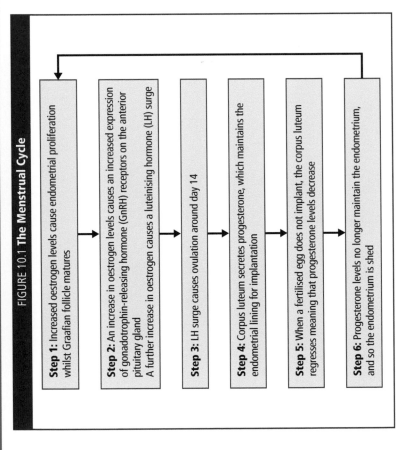

Figure 10.1 The Menstrual Cycle

FIGURE 10.1 **The Menstrual Cycle**

Step 1: Increased oestrogen levels cause endometrial proliferation whilst Graafian follicle matures

Step 2: An increase in oestrogen levels causes an increased expression of gonadotrophin-releasing hormone (GnRH) receptors on the anterior pituitary gland
A further increase in oestrogen causes a luteinising hormone (LH) surge

Step 3: LH surge causes ovulation around day 14

Step 4: Corpus luteum secretes progesterone, which maintains the endometrial lining for implantation

Step 5: When a fertilised egg does not implant, the corpus luteum regresses meaning that progesterone levels decrease

Step 6: Progesterone levels no longer maintain the endometrium, and so the endometrium is shed

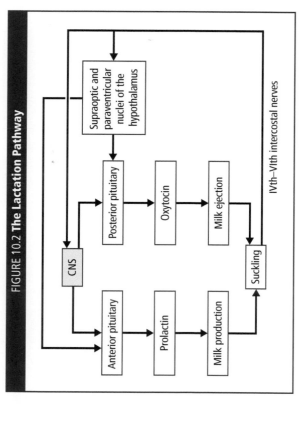

FIGURE 10.2 **The Lactation Pathway**

Supraoptic and paraventricular nuclei of the hypothalamus

Posterior pituitary

Oxytocin

Milk ejection

IVth–VIth intercostal nerves

CNS

Anterior pituitary

Prolactin

Milk production

Suckling

MATERNAL CHANGES DURING PREGNANCY

Respiratory system
- Elevated diaphragm by 4 cm.
- ↓ Expiratory reserve volume.
- ↑ Tidal volume.

Cardiovascular system
- ↓ BP because progesterone decreases vascular resistance by increasing spiral artery formation.
- ↑ Cardiac output.
- ↑ Blood volume since renin–angiotensin–aldosterone system (RAAS) is stimulated by lowered BP.
- Constriction of peripheral circulation (this is why some pregnant women experience Raynaud's phenomenon).

Renal system
- ↑ Kidney size.
- ↑ Frequency of urination.
- ↑ Glomerular filtration rate (GFR).
- ↑ Urinary tract infection risk due to dilated, elongated ureters.

Musculoskeletal system
- Gait changes.
- Lower back pain.
- Ligaments soften.
- Symphysis pubis dysfunction.

MASTITIS

What is mastitis?
This is inflammation of the breast tissue.

Causes
Milk stasis or overproduction causes regional infection of the breast parenchyma with *Staphylococcus aureus*, which enters the breast via trauma to the nipple. This in turn causes mastitis.

Signs and symptoms
- Calor, dolor, rubor and tumour (heat, pain, redness and swelling) of the breast tissue.
- Nipple discharge.
- Fever.

Investigations
- This is a clinical diagnosis.

Treatment
- Conservative: patient education. Encourage mother to continue breastfeeding since this will help to overcome the obstruction.
- Medical: flucloxacillin.

MAP 10.2 **Pregnancy and Lactation**

Dermatology

- Linea nigra.
- Palmar erythema.
- Spider angioma.

Gastrointestinal system

- Constipation.
- Gastro-oesophageal reflux disease.
- ↑ Risk of gallstones.
- Gestational diabetes.

Reproductive system

- ↑ Uterus size.
- Thickening of uterine ligaments.
- Softening of cervix.
- ↑ Vaginal secretions.

Immune system

- Weakened.

Map 10.2 Pregnancy and Lactation

Table 10.1 Commonly Asked about Breast Tumours

TABLE 10.1 Commonly Asked about Breast Tumours

Breast tumour	Benign or malignant	Characteristics	Investigations	Treatment	Complications
Fibroadenoma	Benign	Small Also known as 'breast mouse' due to tumour not being tethered Sharp edges Most common type of benign breast tumour in young women	Undergo triple assessment: 1 Examination 2 Imaging 3 Biopsy Physical examination for lumps and masses Bloods: FBC, WCC, U&Es, LFTs, TFTs	Treatment depends on the cause of the breast tumour and whether it is benign or malignant; treatment may be split into 3 modalities: 1 Conservative: patient and family education; refer to Macmillan nurses; offer genetic counselling; provide psychological assessment and support 2 Medical: prognosis of disease is assessed using the Nottingham Prognostic Index (NPI):	Death Metastasis Complications of chemotherapy regimen Complications of radiotherapy regimen Depression
Intraductal papilloma	Benign	Small Under areola Bloody discharge from nipple	Radiology: mammogram, ultrasound scan, fine needle biopsy under ultrasound guidance (core needle biopsy may be required). Look for metastasis with CXR, CT scan and MRI	$NPI = (0.2 \times \text{invasive size})$ + lymph node stage + grade of tumour	
Phyllodes tumour	Generally benign but has malignant potential	Large Leaf-like projections Rapid growing		Medical therapy may be split into adjuvant hormone therapy, chemotherapy or HER2 directed therapy, depending on the type of tumour	
Ductal carcinoma in situ (DCIS)	Malignant	From ductal hyperplasia Cheesy discharge, confined to ducts	Risk factors for breast cancer: • Female • Increasing age • Family history of breast cancer		
Comedocarcinoma	Malignant	High-grade DCIS Characterised by central necrosis Cheesy discharge			

Table 10.1 Commonly Asked about Breast Tumours

Invasive ductal	Malignant	A hard mass
		Sharp edges
		Most common
		Very aggressive
			• Genetic involvement, e.g. *BRCA1* (chromosome 17) and *BRCA2* (chromosome 13)
			• Alcohol
			• Obesity
			• Increased oestrogen exposure, e.g.:
			  ○ Early menarche
			  ○ Late menopause
			  ○ Oral contraceptive pill use
			  ○ Hormone replacement therapy
			  ○ Decreased parity
			  ○ Not breastfeeding
				Hormone treatment: premenopausal women are treated with tamoxifen (a selective oestrogen receptor modulator); postmenopausal women are treated with anastrazole (an aromatase inhibitor). This is because trials such as the ATAC trial have suggested that aromatase inhibitors are superior to tamoxifen in postmenopausal women. If a woman becomes menopausal during treatment she will benefit from switching medications Chemotherapy and radiotherapy regimens: vary depending on tumour type

Invasive lobular	Malignant	Bilateral presentation		
Medullary	Malignant	Well differentiated Lacks desmoplastic reaction Lymphatic infiltrate Good prognosis		
Inflammatory	Malignant	Invades the dermis and lymphatic system Peau d'orange appearance Retracted nipple		
Paget's disease of the breast	Malignant	Epidermal infiltration of ductal carcinoma Eczematoid nipple changes		

Continued overleaf

Table 10.1 Commonly Asked about Breast Tumours

TABLE 10.1 **Commonly Asked about Breast Tumours** (*Continued*)

Breast tumour	Benign or malignant	Characteristics	Investigations	Treatment	Complications
				HER2 directed therapy: treatment with trastuzumab. This is a monoclonal antibody against the extracellular domain of the HER2 receptor 3 Surgical: the primary aim of surgery is to remove the invasive and non-invasive cancer with clear margins. Lumpectomy followed by a radiotherapy regimen has been shown to be as effective as mastectomy, but mastectomy may be recommended in certain circumstances such as multifocal breast disease. The ipsilateral axilla should also be assessed with ultrasound, fine needle aspiration or core biopsy.	

The Reproductive System

				Clinical staging of the axilla should also be assessed by sentinel lymph node biopsy. The reason for this is to avoid unnecessary axillary clearance in patients

Table 10.1 Commonly Asked about Breast Tumours

Table 10.2 Benign Breast Disease

TABLE 10.2 **Benign Breast Disease**

Benign breast disease	Characteristics	Investigations	Treatment
Mastalgia	Very common Can be cyclical and occurs predominantly in reproductive years Breast cancer often does not present with breast pain Risk factors include: OCP, HRT, pregnancy, increased caffeine intake	Women >35 years typically have a mammogram that is usually normal USS of area of areas of nodularity +/- biopsy	There is no definitive treatment available for breast pain. Options include reducing caffeine intake, decreasing dietary fat, danazol, tamoxifen
Fibroadenoma	Considered as an aberration of normal development. Peak incidence is in the third decade. Discrete, highly mobile, non-tethered and smooth lesions. Also known as 'breast mouse disease' Develops from a lobule in the breast and demonstrates high levels of oestrogen and sulphates. These are usually solitary but sometimes patients present with multiple lesions	Mammogram – popcorn calcification in association with a soft-tissue mass is pathognomonic for fibroadenoma USS +/- biopsy	Usually watchful waiting. If very large may proceed to surgical excision
Phyllodes tumour	Tumours that are on a spectrum from benign to malignant and often clinically mimic a fibroadenoma. Leaf-like projections	Mammogram – calcification is rarely seen, unlike fibroadenomas USS +/- biopsy	Surgical excision due to malignant potential
Hamartomas	Rare. Patients present with a discrete mobile lesion. Hamartomas may be impalpable and an incidental finding on screening mammography	Mammogram – "breast within a breast' appearance with a capsule USS +/- biopsy	Leave alone

Cysts	Common. Peak incidence in 5th–6th decade. Can be single or multiple. They may be completely asymptomatic, detected on screening mammogram or become tender, painful or infected. Patients may present with well-circumscribed, discrete, mobile lesions	Mammogram USS	Aspiration
Duct ectasia	In this benign condition there is a loss of elastin in the ducts and this is associated with chronic inflammatory cell infiltrate. The patient presents with cheesy nipple discharge	Mammogram USS +/– biopsy The above is to exclude any underlying malignancy	Patient reassurance. If troublesome discharge then total duct excision with nipple eversion
Mammary duct fistula	A fistula is an abnormal communication between two epithelial surfaces. Here it is an abnormal connection between the subareolar duct and the skin. This typically occurs in the periaerolar region following periductal mastitis. It is more common in smokers	USS	Antibiotic therapy as per local trust guidelines if in the presence of infection Surgical options include complete duct excision with excision of mammary-duct fistula
Solitary intraductal papilloma	Benign lesion arising from a single central duct. Patients present with spontaneous nipple discharge Conversely, multiple papillomas typically occur in peripheral ducts and patient presents with a palpable mass associated rarely with nipple discharge. They are associated with an increased risk of subsequent ipsilateral breast carcinoma	Mammogram USS +/– biopsy	Duct excision Long-term follow-up with mammogram screening in patients with multiple papillomas

Table 10.2 Benign Breast Disease

Map 10.3 Breast Cancer

What is breast cancer?

Breast cancer arises in the terminal duct-lobular unit. It affects 1 in 8 women in the UK and there are 55,000 women who are diagnosed with breast cancer each year in the UK. The most common type of breast malignancy is invasive ductal carcinoma not otherwise specified (NOS).

Causes

The exact cause and sequencing of breast cancer are incompletely understood. However, there are several risk factors, which are detailed below.

- Genetic risk factors:
  ○ *BRCA1* (chromosome 17).
  ○ *BRCA2* (chromosome 13).
  ○ Cowden syndrome (*PTEN* mutation).
  ○ Li–Fraumeni syndrome (*TP53* mutation).
  ○ Peutz–Jeghers syndrome (*STK11/LKB1* mutation chromosome 19).
  ○ Breast cancer and gastric cancer (*CDH1* mutation).
- The Gail Model for Breast Cancer Risk estimates the absolute 5-year risk and lifetime risk of developing breast cancer. Includes age, age at menarche, age at first live birth, family history of breast cancer, previous breast biopsies, race/ethnicity.
- Others: female, family history, alcohol use, smoking history, nulliparity, not breastfeeding, OCP, HRT.

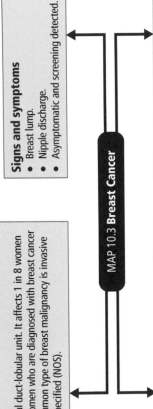

MAP 10.3 Breast Cancer

Signs and symptoms

- Breast lump.
- Nipple discharge.
- Asymptomatic and screening detected.

Investigations

- All patients undergo triple assessment, which includes:
  ○ Examination.
  ○ Imaging.
  ○ Biopsy.
- +/– staging of the axilla.
- Patients are discussed at MDT with their results including receptor status, i.e. ER/PR/Her2.
- +/– CT and MRI looking for metastases.

Prognosis of disease can be assessed using the Nottingham Prognostic Index (NPI):

NPI = (0.2 × invasive size) + lymph node stage + grade of tumour.

TABLE 10.3 TNM for Breast Cancer

	Stage	Primary tumour (T)*	Regional lymph node status (L)	Distant metastasis (M)
T – Tumour	0	TiS	N0	M0
T1	I	T1	N0	M0
Tumour ≤2 cm		T0	N1	M0
T2	IIA	T1	N1	M0
Tumour ≥2 cm but ≥5 cm		T2	N0	M0
T3				
Tumour ≥5 cm				
T4	IIB	T2	N1	M0
Tumour of any size with direct extension to chest wall or skin		T3	N0	M0
N – Lymph node	IIIA	T0	N2	M0
N0		T1	N2	M0
No cancer in regional node		T2	N2	M0
N1		T3	N1/N2	M0
Regional moveable metastasis	IIIB	T4	Any N	M0
N2	IIIC	Any T	N3	M0
Non-movable regional metastases	IV	Any T	Any N	M1
N3				
Cancer in the internal mammary lymph nodes				
M – Metastasis				
M0				
No distant metastases				
M1				
Distant metastases				

Criteria for staging breast tumours according to the UICC ICD-10 TNM classification. *Size measurements are for the tumour's greatest dimension. *Continued overleaf*

213 **The Reproductive System**

Table 10.3 TNM for Breast Cancer

Table 10.3 TNM for Breast Cancer

TABLE 10.3 **TNM for Breast Cancer** (*Continued*)

Treatment

- Conservative: patient and family education, involve breast cancer specialist nurses, refer to Macmillan nurses, referral to fertility services, provide psychological assessment and support, offer genetic counselling, e.g. for *BRCA1* and *BRCA2* pathway.
  - Refer those with unilateral breast cancer <30 years old, bilateral breast cancer <50 years old, those <60 years old with triple-negative breast cancer, male breast cancer at any age, those with non-mucinous ovarian cancer at any age, breast cancer in a patient <45 years old who has a first-degree relative with breast cancer <45 years old, a patient with Ashkenazi Jewish ancestry and breast cancer, patients with a pathology adjusted Manchester score >15.
- Medical: hormonal therapy, Her2 directed therapy and chemo/radiotherapy.
  - Hormone treatment:
    - Tamoxifen: a selective oestrogen receptor modulator (SERM). It has antioestrogen affects in the breast but oestrogenic effects in the uterus and liver. Side effects: endometrial cancer, DVT, PE, hepatotoxicity. Premenopausal women are treated with tamoxifen and postmenopausal women are treated with anastrazole/letrozole (aromatase inhibitors). This is because trials such as the ATAC trial have suggested that aromatase inhibitors are superior to tamoxifen in postmenopausal women. If a woman becomes menopausal during treatment, she will benefit from switching medications.
    - Letrozole: an aromatase inhibitor. Prevents conversion of oestrogens in the peripheral fat. Side effects: arthralgia, fatigue, perimenopausal symptoms such as hot flushes and sweating. Osteoporosis with long-term use. Therefore, patients are often commenced on bone protective agents such as bisphosphonates.
  - Her2 directed therapy:
    - Trastuzumab: a monoclonal antibody. The Her2 gene (tyrosine kinase protein) is amplified up to 30% in breast cancer that is Her2 positive. Trastuzumab targets Her2 causing an immune-mediated response that causes internalisation and recycling for Her2. The Her2 pathway promotes cellular growth. Side effects: fever, cough, headaches, poor sleep, rash, cardiotoxicity, heart failure, allergic reactions.
  - Chemo/radiotherapy: the precise regimen is discussed with an oncology specialist. Chemotherapy and radiotherapy regimens vary depending on tumour type. Clips are placed with the cavity after wide local excision procedures for targeted postoperative radiotherapy. Chemotherapy can be adjuvant or neoadjuvant. Some regimens used are as follows:
    - AC (doxorubicin and cyclophosphamide).
    - EC (epirubicin and cyclophosphamide).
    - AC or EC followed by T (paclitaxel or docetaxel, or the reverse).
    - CAF (cyclophosphamide, doxorubicin and 5-FU).

- Surgical: the primary aim of surgery is to remove the invasive and non-invasive cancer with clear margins. Surgery offered depends on the type of cancer, the location within the breast, the degree of spread, whether the axillary lymph nodes are involved, the tumour to breast size ratio, patient preference and whether plastic surgery reconstructive options are being considered immediately or later. Some examples of procedures are listed below but the ultimate decision is taken at the surgical MDT in line with the patient's oncology results and preferences. Clinical staging of the axilla should also be assessed by sentinel lymph node biopsy. The reason for this is to avoid unnecessary axillary clearance in patients.
  - Wide local excision +/− sentinel lymph node biopsy.
  - Wide local excision +/− axillary node clearance.
  - Radical or simple mastectomy +/− sentinel lymph node biopsy.
  - Radical or simple mastectomy +/− axillary node clearance.
  - Oncoplastic procedures, e.g. therapeutic mammoplasty +/− sentinel lymph node biopsy.
  - Reconstruction options include but are not limited to:
    - Implants.
    - Tissue flap procedures, e.g. transverse rectus abdominis muscle (TRAM) flap, deep inferior epigastric artery perforator (DIEP) flap, latissimus dorsi flap.

Complications

- Death.
- Metastasis – brain, bone, liver, lungs.
- Depression.
- Side effects of treatment.

Table 10.3 TNM for Breast Cancer

TABLE 10.4 Breast Cancer

TABLE 10.4 **Breast Cancer**

Breast cancer	Characteristics
Lobular carcinoma in situ	Proliferative lesion confined to the lobules +/- terminal ductal lobular unit Tends to be an incidental diagnosis Increased risk of multicentric breast cancer This increased risk is distributed evenly between both breasts
Ductal carcinoma in situ	Abnormal proliferation of mammary epithelium that has not invaded the basement membrane. It is the precursor to invasive ductal carcinoma It is a heterogenous group of lesions including several different types, e.g. comedo, cribriform, papillary, micropapillary and solid Microcalcifications are seen on mammogram
Invasive ductal carcinoma	The most common type of breast malignancy. Graded based on tubular formation, nuclear hyperchromatism, mitotic rate and differentiation: 1 = well differentiated; 2 = intermediate; 3 = poorly differentiated
Invasive lobular carcinoma	Malignant transformation of lobular epithelium. It has invaded the breast stroma
Inflammatory	Invades the dermis and lymphatic system. Peau d'orange appearance. Retracted nipple
Paget's disease of the breast	Epidermal infiltration of ductal carcinoma. Eczematoid nipple changes

What is BPH?

This is a benign enlargement of the prostate gland, particularly in the transitional zone. It is common with increasing age.

Causes

There is hypertrophy of the epithelial and stromal cells of the prostate gland.

This classically occurs in the transitional zone of the prostate gland and is thought to be driven by the androgen dihydrotestosterone.

Signs and symptoms
Remember **FUN BOO**:

- **F**requency.
- **U**rgency.
- **N**octuria.
- Those of **B**ladder **O**utflow **O**bstruction (**BOO**):
  - ○ **H**esitancy.
  - ○ Intermittent flow/poor urine stream/ dribbling.
  - ○ Incomplete bladder emptying.

Investigations

- Per rectum (PR) examination: an enlarged but smooth prostate gland with a palpable midline sulcus.
- Urine dipstick, microscopy and culture.
- Bloods: FBCs, U&Es and creatinine (renal function), LFTs.
- Prostate specific antigen (PSA) – usually raised.
- Radiology: ultrasound scan of the urinary tract, transrectal ultrasound scan.

Management

- Conservative: watchful waiting is usually adopted in mild disease.
- Completion of the International Prostate Symptom Score (IPSS). Completion of a voiding diary to see if patient is bothered by their symptoms.
- Medical:
  - ○ α₁-adrenoreceptor blockers, e.g. tamsulosin.
  - ○ 5α-reductase inhibitors, e.g. finasteride.
- Surgical:
  - ○ Transurethral resection of the prostate (TURP).

Complications

- Urinary retention.
- Recurrent urinary tract infections.
- Impaired renal function.
- Haematuria.

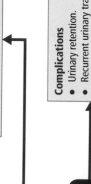

MAP 10.4 **Benign Prostatic Hyperplasia (BPH)**

Map 10.4 Benign Prostatic Hyperplasia (BPH)

Figure 10.3 Zones of the Prostate Gland

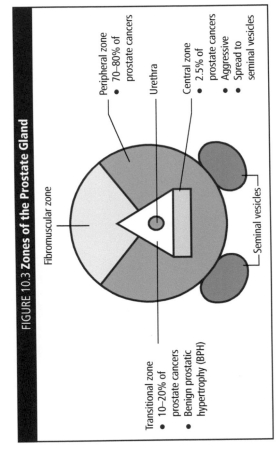

FIGURE 10.3 **Zones of the Prostate Gland**

Fibromuscular zone

Peripheral zone
- 70–80% of prostate cancers

Urethra

Central zone
- 2.5% of prostate cancers
- Aggressive
- Spread to seminal vesicles

Transitional zone
- 10–20% of prostate cancers
- Benign prostatic hypertrophy (BPH)

Seminal vesicles

Investigations

- Per rectum (PR) examination: an enlarged prostate gland that may be uninodular or multinodular. The midline sulcus is usually no longer palpable.
- Urine dipstick, microscopy and culture.
- Bloods: FBCs, U&Es and creatinine (renal function), LFTs.
- Prostate specific antigen (PSA) – usually raised.
- Radiology: transrectal ultrasound and biopsy. If this procedure diagnoses a malignancy then the patient should be sent for an MRI and bone scan to look for distant metastases. Prostate cancer is staged using the TMN system. Since there may also be symptoms of BOO an ultrasound scan of the urinary tract may also be required.

Management

- Conservative: involvement of Macmillan nurses and psychological support.
- Medical:
  - ○ Radiotherapy.
  - ○ Brachytherapy.
  - ○ Goserelin – a luteinising hormone-releasing hormone (LHRH) agonist.
  - ○ Antiandrogens, e.g. cyproterone.
- Surgical:
  - ○ Laparoscopic radical prostatectomy.
  - ○ Transurethral resection of the prostate (TURP).

MAP 10.5 Prostate Cancer

Complications

- Metastasis.
- Death.
- Urinary incontinence.
- Erectile dysfunction.

What is prostate cancer?

This is usually an adenocarcinoma that arises from the peripheral zone of the prostate gland.

Risk factors

- Increasing age.
- Family history of prostate cancer.
- More common in African populations.

Signs and symptoms

- Those of benign prostatic hyperplasia – **FUN BOO** (see page 217).
- Those of metastatic disease:
  - ○ Weight loss.
  - ○ Malaise and fatigue.
  - ○ Usually spreads to bone, therefore bone pain, pathological fracture.

Chapter Eleven Embryology

Map 11.1 Fertilisation

MAP 11.1 **Fertilisation**

The germ layers and their derivatives
- Ectoderm → epidermis, nervous system.
- Mesoderm → muscles, bones connective tissue.
- Endoderm → other organs, e.g. GIT, respiratory tract.

Important dates to remember
- Day 6: implantation.
- Day 9:
  ○ Blastocyst embedded in the endometrium.
  ○ Lacunae formation.
- Day 15: gastrulation.

FIGURE 11.1 Development of the Embryo

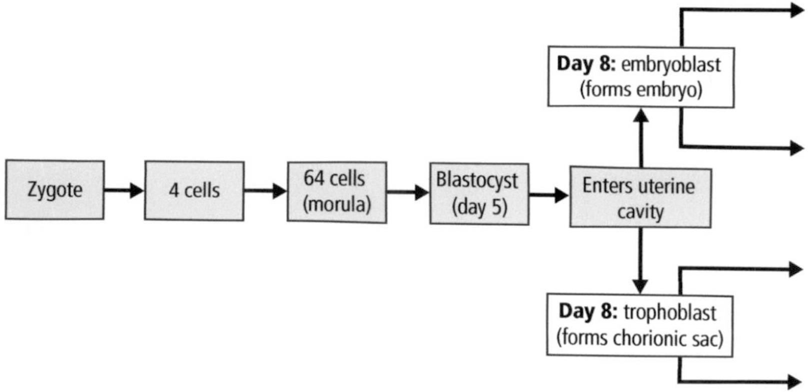

Hypoblast
- Exocoelomic membrane (Heuser's membrane)
- The hypoblast and exocoelomic membrane form the yolk sac

Epiblast
- The small cavity within the epiblast is the amniotic cavity which fills with amniotic fluid
- Amniotic fluid acts as a shock absorber and serves to regulate fetal temperature

Syncytiotrophoblast
- No distinct cell boundaries
- Creates enzymes during implantation

Cytotrophoblast
- Distinct cell boundaries
- Between embryoblast and syncytiotrophoblast

Zygote → 4 cells → 64 cells (morula) → Blastocyst (day 5) → Enters uterine cavity

Day 8: embryoblast (forms embryo)

Day 8: trophoblast (forms chorionic sac)

Figure 11.1 Development of the Embryo

Map 11.2 The Heart

Development of the heart

- Develops during week 3 from cardiac progenitor cells.
- The heart tube forms from 2 endocardial tubes at day 21 and the heart begins to beat on day 22.
- Note that blood flows through the endocardial tube caudocranially:
  ○ Truncus arteriosus → aorta and pulmonary trunk.
  ○ Bulbus cordis → smooth part of right ventricle (conus arteriosus); smooth part of left ventricle (aortic vestibule).
  ○ Primitive ventricle → trabeculated part of right and left ventricles.
  ○ Primitive atrium → trabeculated part of right and left atrium.
  ○ Sinus venosus → smooth part of right atrium, coronary sinus, oblique vein of left atrium.
- The ventricle grows at a faster rate than the other areas causing the cardiac loop to fold in a U shape.
- The cardiac septa form between the 27th and 37th day.

Cardiovascular teratogens

Remember **RAT**:

- **R**etinoic acid, **R**ubella virus.
- **A**lcohol.
- **T**halidomide.

MAP 11.2 The Heart

Molecular regulation

- NKX-2.5: induces heart formation and also plays a role in expression of *HAND 1* and *HAND 2*, which are important regulators of ventricle differentiation.
- Wnt inhibitors.
- Bone morphogenetic proteins BMP-2 and BMP-4 along with Wnt inhibitors are responsible for NKX-2.5 expression.
- Laterality-inducing genes *NODAL* and *LEFTY2* cause *PITX2* expression: plays a role in cardiac loop formation.

Examples of defects

- Atrial septal defect (ASD): ostium secundum defect.
- Ostium primum defect.
- Tricuspid atresia.
- Ebstein's anomaly.
- Ventricular septal defect (VSD).
- Tetralogy of Fallot (ToF):
  ○ Pulmonary stenosis.
  ○ Overriding aorta.
  ○ VSD.
  ○ Right ventricular hypertrophy.
- Transposition of the great vessels.
- Persistent truncus arteriosus.

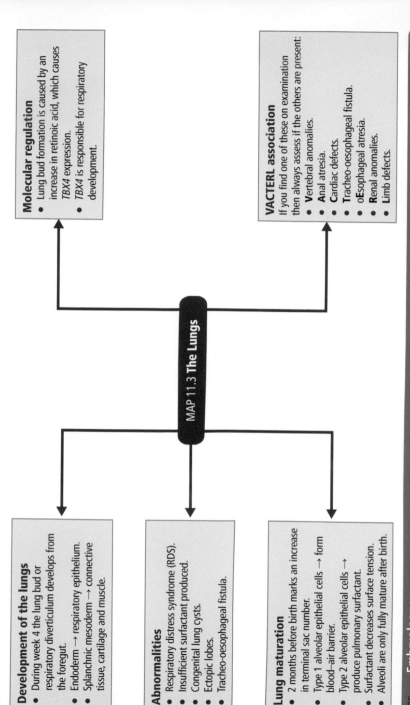

Molecular regulation

- Lung bud formation is caused by an increase in retinoic acid, which causes *TBX4* expression.
- *TBX4* is responsible for respiratory development.

VACTERL association

If you find one of these on examination then always assess if the others are present:

- **V**ertebral anomalies.
- **A**nal atresia.
- **C**ardiac defects.
- **T**racheo-oesophageal fistula.
- o**E**sophageal atresia.
- **R**enal anomalies.
- **L**imb defects.

MAP 11.3 The Lungs

Development of the lungs

- During week 4 the lung bud or respiratory diverticulum develops from the foregut.
- Endoderm → respiratory epithelium.
- Splanchnic mesoderm → connective tissue, cartilage and muscle.

Abnormalities

- Respiratory distress syndrome (RDS).
- Insufficient surfactant produced.
- Congenital lung cysts.
- Ectopic lobes.
- Tracheo-oesophageal fistula.

Lung maturation

- 2 months before birth marks an increase in terminal sac number.
- Type 1 alveolar epithelial cells → form blood–air barrier.
- Type 2 alveolar epithelial cells → produce pulmonary surfactant.
- Surfactant decreases surface tension.
- Alveoli are only fully mature after birth.

Map 11.3 The Lungs

Map 11.4 The Gastrointestinal Tract (GIT)

Development of the GIT

There are 4 parts to the primitive gut. These are the:

1 pharyngeal gut
2 foregut
3 midgut
4 hindgut.

- Endoderm → epithelial lining, pancreatic endocrine glands, pancreatic exocrine glands and hepatocytes.
- Visceral mesoderm → connective tissue and muscle.

MAP 11.4
The Gastrointestinal Tract (GIT)

Molecular regulation

Region of GIT	Gene involved
Oesophagus	SOX-2
Stomach	SOX-2
Small intestine	CDXC HOX9–10
Caecum	HOX9–11
Large intestine	CDXA HOX9–12
Cloaca	HOX9–13
Rectum	CDXA
Liver	HOX
Duodenum	PDX1

Sonic hedgehog (SHH) gene causes epithelial–mesenchymal interaction and HOX gene expression.

Abnormalities

- Oesophageal atresia.
- Congenital hiatus hernia.
- Pyloric stenosis.
- Accessory hepatic ducts.
- Duplication of gallbladder.
- Extrahepatic biliary atresia.
- Annular pancreas.
- Omphalocoele.
- Gastroschisis.
- Rectourethral fistula.
- Rectovaginal fistula.
- Hirschsprung's disease.

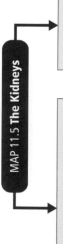

MAP 11.5 The Kidneys

Development of the kidneys

3 sets of kidneys form during development:

1 Pronephros: non-functional
2 Mesonephros: semi-functional
3 Metanephros: permanent kidneys.

The kidneys develop from intermediate mesoderm.

Abnormalities

- Autosomal recessive polycystic kidney disease (ARPKD).
- Autosomal dominant polycystic kidney disease (ADPKD).
- Wilms' tumour.
- Denys–Drash syndrome.
- Renal agenesis.
- Pelvic kidney.
- Horseshoe kidney.

FIGURE 11.2 Molecular Regulation of Kidney Development

```
              WT1
               ↓
        Ureteric bud formation
         ↙              ↘
Mesenchyme induction via:    Nephron formation via:
• FGF2                       • WNT9B
• BMP7                       • WNT6
                             • PAX2
                             • WNT4
```

FIGURE 11.3 Kidney Development

```
Mesonephric bud → Ureteric bud → Renal pelvis → Cranial and caudal major calyces → 2 × buds → 12+ generations → Minor calyces
```

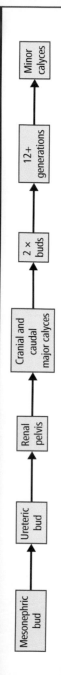

Map 11.5 The Kidneys

Embryology

Figure 11.4 Brain Development

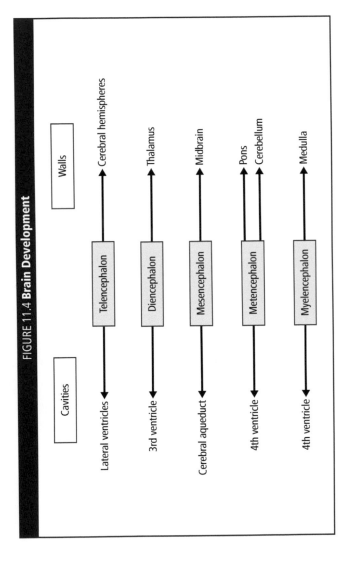

FIGURE 11.4 **Brain Development**

MAP 11.6 Genital Development

Development of the male and female reproductive systems
- From intermediate mesoderm.
- Male gender is determined by sex-determining region on Y chromosome (*SRY* gene).
- Without *SRY* gene expression the embryo is female.

Abnormalities
- Androgen insensitivity syndrome.
- Congenital adrenal hyperplasia.
- Hermaphroditism.
- Vaginal agenesis.
- Ambiguous genitalia.
- Intersex syndromes.
- Cryptorchidism.
- Hypospadias.

Molecular development
- Male: *SRY* gene → SOX9 → SP1 → testes.
- Female: *WNT4* → DAX1 → ovaries.

Figure 11.5 Development of the Reproductive System

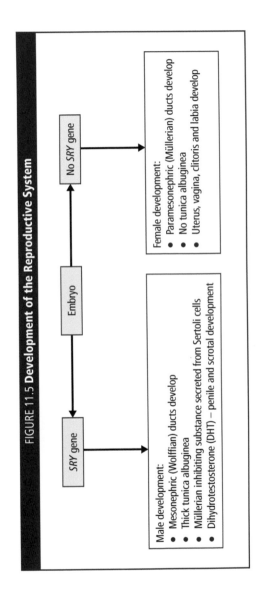

FIGURE 11.5 **Development of the Reproductive System**

Male development:
- Mesonephric (Wolffian) ducts develop
- Thick tunica albuginea
- Müllerian inhibiting substance secreted from Sertoli cells
- Dihydrotestosterone (DHT) – penile and scrotal development

Female development:
- Paramesonephric (Müllerian) ducts develop
- No tunica albuginea
- Uterus, vagina, clitoris and labia develop

Map 12.1 X-Linked Recessive Disorders

HAEMOPHILIA A
What is haemophilia A?
This is an X-linked recessive bleeding and bruising disorder.

Causes
- Deficiency of factor VIII.

Signs and symptoms
These vary depending on disease severity. Bleeding is the main feature and this is prolonged, resulting in the need for investigations to uncover the cause. Positive family history may tailor diagnosis.

Investigations
- Low factor VIII levels: the lower the level, the more severe the disease.
- Coagulation factor assay.
- Increased PTT but normal PT.

Treatment
- Conservative: patient and parent education. Genetic counselling and testing are now available. Avoid anticoagulant medication, e.g. nonsteroidal anti-inflammatory drugs (NSAIDs), warfarin, aspirin.
- Medical:
  - Mild: desmopressin.
  - Severe: require IV replacement with plasma concentrate factor VIII.

Complications
- Patient's immune system may start to reject the IV plasma concentrate factor VIII by making inhibitors.
- Joint destruction by recurrent bleeding.

MAP 12.1 **X-Linked Recessive Disorders**

HAEMOPHILIA B
What is haemophilia B?
Haemophilia B, also known as Christmas disease, is an X-linked recessive bleeding and bruising disorder.

Causes
- Deficiency of factor IX.

Signs and symptoms
These vary depending on disease severity. Bleeding is the main feature of this disease and this is prolonged, resulting in the need for tests to uncover the cause. Positive family history may tailor diagnosis.

Investigations
- Low factor IX levels: the lower the level, the more severe the disease.
- Coagulation factor assay.
- Increased PTT but normal PT.

Treatment
- Conservative: patient and parent education. Genetic counselling and testing are now available. Avoid anticoagulant medication, e.g. NSAIDs, warfarin, aspirin.
- Medical: IV infusion of factor IX.

Complications
- Joint destruction by recurrent bleeding.

Continued overleaf

Map 12.1 X-Linked Recessive Disorders

233   **Genetic Disorders**

Map 12.2   X-Linked Recessive Disorders

DUCHENNE MUSCULAR DYSTROPHY

What is Duchenne muscular dystrophy?

This is a form of muscular dystrophy.

Causes

- Mutated dystrophin gene at locus Xp21.

Signs and symptoms

- Patient falls frequently.
- Fatigue.
- Toe walking/difficulty walking.
- Muscle weakness.
- Muscle pseudohypertrophy.
- Muscle fibrosis.
- Positive Gower's test.

Investigations

- DNA testing: confirms mutation of dystrophin gene.
- Creatine phosphokinase test. Results show increased levels.
- Muscle biopsy: confirms mutation of dystrophin gene.
- Electromyography (EMG): analyses muscle destruction.

Treatment

There is no specific treatment for this disease. Prednisolone and creatinine replacement may be considered. Patient will be wheelchair bound at ~12 years; refer to occupational therapy and physiotherapy. Patient and parent education and support are essential since this condition is very debilitating and life expectancy is ~25–30 years.

Complications

- Scoliosis.
- Respiratory complications and increased risk of respiratory infections.
- Cardiomyopathy.
- Osteoporosis.

MAP 12.2 **X-Linked Recessive Disorders** (*Continued*)

LESCH–NYHAN SYNDROME

What is Lesch–Nyhan syndrome?

This is a rare X-linked recessive disorder that causes a build-up of uric acid in the body.

Causes
- Deficiency of hypoxanthine–guanine phosphoribosyltransferase (HGPRT).

Signs and symptoms
- Behavioural problems.
- Intellectual impairment.
- Self-harming behaviour.
- Poor muscle control.
- Symptoms of gout, see page 161.

Investigations
- Bloods: FBC, U&Es, LFTs, creatinine, uric acid, HGPRT.
- Radiology: ultrasound scan of kidneys for radiolucent urate renal calculi.

Treatment
- Conservative: parent education.
- Medical: allopurinol (to decrease uric acid levels). For neurological and behavioural problems consider benzodiazepines and baclofen.

Complications
- Gout.
- Renal calculi.
- Self-harm.

Continued overleaf

RETT'S SYNDROME

What is Rett's syndrome?

This is a neurodevelopmental disorder of brain grey matter.

Causes

- Mutation of the methyl-CpG binding protein-2 (*MECP2*) gene.

Signs and symptoms

- Neurological dysfunction, e.g.:
  - Ataxia.
  - Hypotonia.
  - Inability to walk or altered gait.
  - Chorea.
- Autistic behaviour, e.g.:
  - Lack of eye contact.
  - Lack of theory of mind.
  - Decreased social interaction.
  - Speech deficit.
  - Screaming.

Investigations

- DNA sequencing of *MECP2* gene is diagnostic.

Treatment

- Conservative: parent education.
- Medical: treatment of complications.

AICARDI'S SYNDROME

What is Aicardi's syndrome?

This is an X-linked recessive condition in which there is partial or complete absence of the corpus callosum. Retinal abnormalities and seizures are also present.

Causes

The exact cause remains unknown but it is thought to be due to new mutations that are passed genetically to offspring via X-linked recessive inheritance.

Signs and symptoms

- Infantile spasms.

Investigations

- Radiology: CT or MRI confirming corpus callosum agenesis.

Treatment

- Conservative: parent education. Referral to speech and language therapy, neuropsychologist, neurology and physiotherapy.
- Medical: there is no specific treatment. Manage epilepsy, see pages 116–121.

Complications

- Hydrocephalus.
- Porencephalic cysts.

MAP 12.3 **X-Linked Recessive Disorders** (*Continued*)

Complications
- Arrhythmias.
- Epilepsy.
- Gastro-oesophageal reflux disease.
- Osteoporosis.

KLINEFELTER'S SYNDROME
What is Klinefelter's syndrome?
This is a syndrome in which males have an extra X chromosome.
Chromosomally, patients are XXY.

Causes
- An additional X chromosome.

Signs and symptoms
- Hypogonadism.
- Long limbs.
- Late onset of puberty.
- Gynaecomastia.
- Infertility.

Investigations
- Prenatal diagnosis.
- Follicle-stimulating hormone (FSH) and luteinising hormone (LH) levels.

Treatment
- Conservative: patient and parent education. Genetic counselling.
- Medical: no specific medical therapy. Treat comorbidities such as depression, which is common in this group.

Complications
- Infertility.
- Depression.

Map 12.3 X-Linked Recessive Disorders

Map 12.4 Autosomal Dominant Conditions

HUNTINGTON'S DISEASE

What is Huntington's disease?

This is an autosomal dominant inherited neurodegenerative disorder.

Causes

- Abnormal *huntingtin* gene on chromosome 4.
- Leads to (CAG)n repeats.
- The longer the (CAG)n repeats, the earlier the onset of disease.

Signs and symptoms

- Present at ~35 years of age.
- Progressive decline in motor coordination.
- Chorea.
- Cognitive decline.
- Personality change.

Investigations

- Genetic testing confirms diagnosis.

Treatment

- Conservative: patient education. Genetic counselling.
- Medical: there is no specific treatment. Manage complications.

Complications

- Chorea.
- Dementia.
- Dysphagia.
- Depression.
- Anxiety.

MAP 12.4 Autosomal
Dominant Conditions

FAMILIAL ADENOMATOUS POLYPOSIS (FAP)

What is FAP?

This is an autosomal dominant condition that causes thousands of polyps to develop in the large intestine. It predisposes patients to colon cancer.

Causes

- Mutation in the *APC* gene on chromosome 5.

Signs and symptoms

- Blood in stool.
- Signs of malignancy, see page 54.

Investigations

See page 54.

- Genetic testing and colonoscopy are diagnostic.

Treatment

- Surgical resection of the affected bowel is the treatment of choice.

Complications

- Colon cancer.

EHLERS–DANLOS SYNDROME

What is Ehlers–Danlos syndrome?

This is a type of connective tissue disorder that results from defective collagen.

Causes

- Defect in type I and type III collagen synthesis.

Signs and symptoms

Remember these as **HBO**:

- **H**yperextension.
- **B**ruise easily.
- **O**steoarthritis (early onset).

Investigations

- Collagen gene mutation testing.
- Skin biopsy for collagen typing.
- ECHO for valvular heart disease and aortic dilation.

Treatment

- Conservative: patient education.
- Medical: there is no specific treatment for this condition. Manage complications.

Complications

- Valvular heart disease.
- Joint deformities, e.g. osteoarthritis and scoliosis.
- Anal prolapse.
- Complications during pregnancy.

Continued overleaf

Map 12.4 Autosomal Dominant Conditions

MAP 12.5 Autosomal Dominant Conditions (Continued)

TUBEROUS SCLEROSIS

What is tuberous sclerosis?

This condition causes non-malignant tumours to grow in a variety of organs.

Causes

- Mutation of *TSC1* and *TSC2* genes. *TSC1* gene codes for hamartin protein. *TCS2* gene codes for tuberin protein.

Signs and symptoms

These depend on where the tumours form. Some examples include:

- Renal angiomyolipomas: haematuria.
- Rhabdomyomas: cardiac arrhythmias.
- Facial angiofibromas: butterfly distribution on face.
- Ash leaf spots.
- Coloboma.

Investigations

- Fundoscopy.
- Examine skin with Wood's lamp for ash leaf spots and angiofibromas.
- Radiology: CT scan, MRI, ECHO (rhabdomyoma), renal ultrasound scan (angiomyolipoma).

MARFAN'S SYNDROME

What is Marfan's syndrome?

This is a disorder of connective tissue due to abnormal fibrillin-1 formation.

Causes

- Mutated *FBN1* gene.

Signs and symptoms

A – Arachnodactyly, Astigmatism, Angina, Aortic Aneurysm/dissection.

B – Bullae, Bronchiectasis.

C – Cyanosis, Cysts (spinal), Coarctation of the aorta.

D – Dolichostenomelia, Dislocation of lens.

P – Pectus carinatum/excavatum, high Palate, Palpitations.

Investigations

- This is a clinical diagnosis.
- ECG and ECHO to monitor cardiac complications.
- MRI of spinal cord to monitor neurological complications.

Treatment

- Conservative: patient education.
- Medical: there is no specific treatment. Manage complications.

Complications

- Renal failure.
- Status epilepticus.
- Sudden unexpected death in epilepsy (SUDEP).

Treatment

- Conservative: patient education. Genetic counselling.
- Medical: there is no specific treatment. Manage complications, e.g. prescribe a beta-blocker (if not contraindicated) to reduce blood pressure.
- Surgery: to manage complications.

Complications

- Aortic dissection/aneurysm.
- Valvular disease.
- Glaucoma.
- Scoliosis.
- Depression.

Map 12.5 Autosomal Dominant Conditions

Map 12.6 Autosomal Recessive Conditions

FRIEDREICH'S ATAXIA
What is Friedreich's ataxia?

This is an autosomal recessive condition that causes neural degeneration.

Causes
- Mutation of *FXN* gene on chromosome 9 causes GAA repeats and abnormal frataxin production.

Signs and symptoms
- Abnormal gait.
- Speech disturbance.
- Cardiomyopathy.

Investigations
- Genetic testing.
- Nerve conduction studies.
- ECG for cardiac complications.
- Vitamin E levels: rule out vitamin E deficiency as a differential diagnosis.

Treatment
- Conservative: patient and parent education. Refer to physiotherapy and speech and language therapy.
- Medical: there is no specific treatment for this condition. Manage complications.

PHENYLKETONURIA
What is phenylketonuria?

This is an autosomal recessive disease in which levels of phenylalanine increase due to the lack of phenylalanine hydroxylase (PAH). Phenylalanine is subsequently converted to phenylpyruvate instead of tyrosine.

Causes
- Mutation in the gene that codes for PAH.

Signs and symptoms
- Asymptomatic at birth.
- Severe learning difficulties.
- Seizures.

Investigations
- Guthrie heel prick test is diagnostic.

Treatment
- Conservative: parent education. Genetic counselling.
- Patients are on lifelong low phenylalanine diet.

Complications
- Neurobehavioural problems.
- Seizures.

MAP 12.6 Autosomal Recessive Conditions

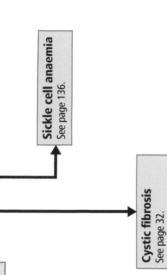

Complications
- Cardiomyopathy.
- Scoliosis.
- Pes cavus (high instep).
- Diabetes mellitus.
- Hearing loss.

Thalassaemia
See page 138.

Sickle cell anaemia
See page 136.

Cystic fibrosis
See page 32.

Map 12.6 Autosomal Recessive Conditions

Map 12.7   Trisomies

DOWN'S SYNDROME

What is Down's syndrome?

Down's syndrome is the most common trisomy abnormality, which is characterised by specific signs and symptoms.

Causes

• Trisomy 21.

Signs and symptoms

• Learning difficulties.
• Short stature.
• Flattened nose.
• Slanted eyes.
• Simian crease.
• Gap between 1st and 2nd toes.

Investigations

• Antenatal testing: ultrasound for nuchal translucency.
• Radiology: pelvic X-ray shows dysplastic pelvis.
• ECG and ECHO for cardiac complications.

Treatment

• Conservative: parent education.
• Medical: management of complications.
• Surgical: management of complications.

Complications

• Atrial septal defects.

EDWARD'S SYNDROME

What is Edward's syndrome?

Edward's syndrome is the second most common trisomy abnormality.

Causes

• Trisomy 18.

Signs and symptoms

• Rocker-bottom feet.
• Learning difficulties.
• Clenched hands.
• Low-set ears.
• Micrognathia.
• Cleft lip or cleft palate.
• Undescended testicles.

Investigations

• Chromosomal analysis confirms diagnosis.
• ECG and ECHO for cardiac complications.

Treatment

• Conservative: parent education and support particularly since life expectancy is 4 months to 1 year.

Complications

• Coarctation of the aorta.
• Atrial septal defects.

MAP 12.7
Trisomies

- Ventricular septal defects.
- Duodenal atresia.
- Acute lymphoblastic leukaemia.
- Alzheimer's disease.
- Hypothyroidism.

- Inguinal hernia.
- Omphalocoele.
- Renal agenesis.

PATAU'S SYNDROME

What is Patau's syndrome?
This is a chromosomal abnormality.

Causes
- Trisomy 13.

Signs and symptoms
- Learning difficulties.
- Congenital heart disease.
- Cleft lip/palate.
- Microcephaly.
- Polydactyly.
- Rocker-bottom feet.

Investigations
- Chromosomal analysis confirms diagnosis.
- ECG and ECHO for cardiac complications.

Treatment
- Conservative: parent education and support particularly since life expectancy is <1 year.

Complications
- Omphalocoele.
- Polycystic kidneys.
- Ventricular septal defects.
- Inguinal hernia.

Map 12.7 Trisomies

Name of criteria	Name of disease
Framingham Criteria	Congestive cardiac failure
New York Heart Association Classification	Heart failure
QRISK Score	Calculates 10-year cardiovascular risk
Duke Criteria	Infective endocarditis
Rockall Risk Scoring Criteria	Upper gastrointestinal bleeding
Rome III Criteria	Irritable bowel syndrome
Alvarado Score	Acute appendicitis
Child–Pugh Grading System	Cirrhosis and risk of variceal bleeding
Truelove and Witts Criteria	Ulcerative colitis
Vienna Criteria	Crohn's disease
Los Angeles Classification	Gastro-oesophageal reflux disease
Amsterdam Criteria	Hereditary nonpolyposis colorectal cancer (HNPCC)
Dukes' Staging System	Colorectal cancer
Rifle Criteria	Acute kidney injury
MRC Classification	Grading for muscle power
McDonald Criteria	Multiple sclerosis
Ann Arbor Staging Classification	Hodgkin's and non-Hodgkin's lymphoma
Psoriasis Area and Severity Index	Psoriasis
Disease Activity in Psoriatic Arthritis Score	Psoriatic arthritis
Beighton Criteria	Joint hypermobility
Cardiac Failure, Hypertension, Age, Diabetes, Stroke system (CHADS2) Score	Calculates risk of stroke in patients with AF

Disease	Page No.	Website
Acute kidney injury	70	https://www.nice.org.uk/guidance/conditions-and-diseases/kidney-conditions/acute-kidney-injury
Acute pancreatitis	56	https://www.nice.org.uk/guidance/ng104
Anaemia	128	https://cks.nice.org.uk/topics/anaemia-iron-deficiency/
Angina pectoris	8	https://www.nice.org.uk/guidance/conditions-and-diseases/cardiovascular-conditions/stable-angina
Asthma	26	https://www.nice.org.uk/guidance/conditions-and-diseases/respiratory-conditions/asthma https://www.brit-thoracic.org.uk/quality-improvement/guidelines/asthma/
Atrial fibrillation	18	https://www.nice.org.uk/guidance/ng196
Breast cancer	212	https://cks.nice.org.uk/topics/breast-cancer-recognition-referral/diagnosis/symptoms-suggestive-of-breast-cancer/
Bronchiectasis	31	https://pathways.nice.org.uk/pathways/bronchiectasis-non-cystic-fibrosis-antimicrobial-prescribing
Cardiovascular disease prevention	6,8	https://pathways.nice.org.uk/pathways/cardiovascular-disease-prevention
Chronic kidney injury	70	https://www.nice.org.uk/guidance/conditions-and-diseases/kidney-conditions/chronic-kidney-disease
Chronic obstructive pulmonary disease	24	https://www.nice.org.uk/guidance/conditions-and-diseases/respiratory-conditions/chronic-obstructive-pulmonary-disease
Colorectal cancer	54	https://www.nice.org.uk/guidance/conditions-and-diseases/cancer/colorectal-cancer
Crohn's disease	46	https://www.nice.org.uk/guidance/ng129
Cushing's syndrome	98	https://www.thelancet.com/journals/landia/article/PIIS2213-8587(21)00235-7/fulltext
Deep vein thrombosis	37	https://pathways.nice.org.uk/pathways/venous-thromboembolism https://www.mdcalc.com/wells-criteria-dvt
Dementia	112	https://cks.nice.org.uk/topics/dementia/

Disease	Page No.	Website
Diabetes mellitus	86	Type 1: https://pathways.nice.org.uk/pathways/type-1-diabetes-in-adults Type 2: https://pathways.nice.org.uk/pathways/type-2-diabetes-in-adults
Epilepsy	116	https://cks.nice.org.uk/topics/epilepsy/
Heart failure	2	https://www.nice.org.uk/guidance/ng106
Hepatitis B	52	https://www.nice.org.uk/guidance/qs65
HIV	190	https://www.bhiva.org/guidelines
Hypertension	16	https://pathways.nice.org.uk/pathways/hypertension/ hypertension-overview#content=view-node: nodes-hypertension-not-diagnosed
Hypothyroidism/ hyperthyroidism	80, 82	https://www.nice.org.uk/guidance/ng145
Infective endocarditis	10	https://pathways.nice.org.uk/pathways/prophylaxis-against-infective-endocarditis
Irritable bowel syndrome	44	https://www.nice.org.uk/guidance/conditions-and-diseases/ digestive-tract-conditions/irritable-bowel-syndrome
Lung cancer	35	https://www.nice.org.uk/guidance/conditions-and-diseases/ cancer/lung-cancer
Malaria	184	https://cks.nice.org.uk/topics/malaria/
Mastitis	204	https://cks.nice.org.uk/topics/mastitis-breast-abscess/
Multiple sclerosis	122	https://cks.nice.org.uk/topics/multiple-sclerosis/
Myocardial infarction	6	https://www.nice.org.uk/guidance/ng185
Osteoarthritis	156	https://cks.nice.org.uk/topics/osteoarthritis/
Osteoporosis	163	https://cks.nice.org.uk/topics/osteoporosis-prevention-of-fragility-fractures/
Parkinson's disease	124	https://cks.nice.org.uk/topics/parkinsons-disease/
Pneumonia	29	https://www.nice.org.uk/guidance/qs110
Pneumothorax	39	https://www.ebm-guidelines.com/ebmg/ltk.free?p_artikkeli=ebm00133
Psoriasis	159	https://cks.nice.org.uk/topics/psoriasis/

Disease	Page No.	Website
Pulmonary embolism	38	https://cks.nice.org.uk/topics/pulmonary-embolism/ https://www.mdcalc.com/wells-criteria-pulmonary-embolism
Rheumatoid arthritis	156	https://cks.nice.org.uk/topics/rheumatoid-arthritis/
Stroke	110	https://cks.nice.org.uk/topics/stroke-tia/
Thyroid cancer	84	https://www.nice.org.uk/guidance/conditions-and-diseases/cancer/thyroid-cancer
Tuberculosis	186	https://cks.nice.org.uk/topics/tuberculosis/
Ulcerative colitis	46	https://www.nice.org.uk/guidance/ng130
Upper GI bleeding	43	https://www.nice.org.uk/guidance/conditions-and-diseases/digestive-tract-conditions/upper-gastrointestinal-bleeding
Urinary tract infection	66	https://www.nice.org.uk/guidance/conditions-and-diseases/urological-conditions/urinary-tract-infection

Index

Index

Index